Simple

Allergy

Friendly

Cookbook

MARIANNE AND DON WEIDEMANN

Simple Allergy Friendly Cookbook

Big Lemon Books
4708 Hoffman Drive
Austin, Texas 78749

www.allergyfreeeats.com

First Edition
First Printing January 2010

ISBN 978-0-9845474-01

Cover design by Don Weidemann

Although information herein is based on the authors' extensive experience
and knowledge, it is not intended to substitute for the services
of medical professionals for treatment and diagnosis.

Printed in the United States of America
at Morgan Printing in Austin, Texas

*This book is dedicated
with all the love we have
to our beautiful daughters,
Jamie and Margot.*

Table of Contents

    Gluten-Free Flour Mix

    Gluten-Free Websites and Gluten-Free All Stars

Foreword

Food Allergies

Food allergies are responsible for as many as half of all health problems in America today. The good news here is that certain foods can be avoided, which allows us a measure of control over our health.

There are two basic types of food allergy reactions. One is a histamine reaction, which can range from rashes or itchy lips (many people experience this with strawberries or melons) to the very serious anaphylactic reactions some people have to peanuts. The other and much more common reaction is an autoimmune reaction such as migraine, arthritis, eczema or colitis caused by MSG, milk, wheat, corn, gluten, etc.

The histamine allergy reactions are easily identified by the immediate onset of symptoms and can be confirmed by standard scratch testing by an allergist. Autoimmune reactions on the other hand are delayed onset (from 15 minutes to days) and cannot be identified by scratch testing. The gold standard for autoimmune reactions is elimination of the specific food item for long enough for the symptoms to subside (from a few days to six months). Then reintroduce the food to see if symptoms recur. The trick is in knowing what to eliminate. Methods range from fasting to eliminating all the common allergens to manual muscle testing to blood typing.

John Bandy, DC.

Preface

This project is the result of two requests. A few years ago while gathered around the Christmas table, our daughters, 21 and 23, talked about how they would like us to leave a legacy for them of the dishes we have shared in the past. A seed was planted. Drawing on shared memories of gatherings in the kitchen, aromas, tastes, conversation and the warmth of family, we began to pull together a few recipes.

A week later at work, a similar request was made by Eleanor McCulley, R.N., Ph.D and Marcia Taylor, RN, L.Ac., two visionaries who daily help others to achieve optimal health. Not only do we work together, we often find ourselves grabbing a quick lunch in our breakroom. They would ask questions about the food I brought in, and were intrigued by the combination of healthy ingredients. Desiring healthy recipes for their clients, they asked if it was possible to compile a handout for their clients.

Realizing this was our opportunity to not only show how easy it is to prepare allergen-free meals, we could also reveal the numerous code words for monosodium glutamate, or MSG. As MSG is known for its damage to the neurological system, we jumped at the chance to make this happen.

You have to know from the start, 90 percent of our meals are cooked by my husband and co-author of this book, Don. He considers the kitchen his playground and food an artform. Beautifully prepared food springs forth in abundance from our kitchen, continually delighting me, and hopefully, now others.

Enjoy!

Marianne Weidemann

Let Us Give Thanks...

To John Bandy for his wisdom and support and his great barbeque sauce recipe. His knowledge of allergies is the foundation for this guide.

To Norma Bandy and John Bandy for their vision of an holistic health center, and opening Austin Holistic Health. Thanks for supporting us with our Simple Allergy Friendly Cookbook.

To the staff at Morgan Printing and especially Terry Sherrell. We are blessed to have good friends in good places. Terry guided us through each phase with great finesse and expertise, inspiring us to keep the momentum. We truly appreciate her time spent bringing our book to fruition.

To Gayle Harris, our dear friend, for her wit, charm and lovely gluten-free snacks. Gayle edited our book, inspired me to keep moving forward, and contributed an award-winning cookie recipe.

To Eleanor McCulley, R.N., PhD., and Marcia Taylor, R.N. L.Ac., who, as clinical nutritionists and NAET practitioners, wanted healthy recipes for their clients. Thanks for their requests which helped shape the book, as well as their support and friendship.

A special thanks to Jack Samuels for his dedication to the cause, truthinlabeling.ORG. This website is dedicated to people with problems that defy medical diagnosis, only to discover that eliminating MSG allows them to be well again.

To all the special friends and family who contributed recipes, love, inspiration and support. Thanks to one and all who continue their love and support for our allergy-free cooking.

Introduction

This book is for everyone. If you have been wondering how you or your family members can get by without gluten, milk, corn, wheat, or just want to eat a clean diet free of MSG and other harmful chemicals, this cookbook will be your guide.

As is often the case, I began my search for good health after my own health crisis. Suffering from constant infections, and no stamina for physical activity, I had lost most of my muscle mass. My goal had become to "get my life back." I wanted to hike and play with my daughters, and have a body that functioned normally. This goal seemed unattainable, as I was going nowhere with traditional medicine, or even alternative health providers.

I must stop and give credit at this point to a very influential person in my life: Shakti Miller, LCSW and naturopath. Along with restoring my health, she directed me toward a more conscious path physically, emotionally and spiritually.

From there, I studied everything my working schedule would allow. After hands-on training from Shakti, gaining a diploma in herbology, a Doctor of Naturopathy degree, and a certification in European Iridology, I wanted to learn more. I became certified in Essential Oil Therapy. Shakti and I traveled several times to Colorado together to study beginning and advanced levels with Hanna Kroeger. (See her website for more information.)

Knowing now, that good health is spiritual, mental, emotional and physical, my everyday aim is to address them all. Although cooking and eating are basically physical activities, there is a certain sense of satisfaction emotionally, mentally, and spiritually, when you sit down to a meal that has been prepared out of love, with nutritious, healthy ingredients. It all adds up to good health.

Common Allergens

Some of the more common genetic allergies are due to the following (see ingredients to avoid for each of these listed under each heading):

- Wheat
- Corn
- Milk
- Cheese
- Gluten

*A note on the MF rating (milk allergy).

If you are allergic to lactalbumin, then you can eat most hard cheeses and butter, and in some cases pure cream (if they have not added in skim milk), because the lactalbumin has been digested by the mold. You may also use milk or milk products in a casserole or pie if cooked at 350°F for one hour, as lactalbumin is heat sensitive.

If you are allergic to casein and lactalbumin, then the entire milk and cheese listing will apply and you will need the DF or dairy free diet.

Definitions of Abbreviations Used in This Book

You will see a combination of these next to each recipe.

If in doubt of any ingredient's safety, go to *www.celicsociety.com/searchCategory.asp*. Select the item in question and this site will tell you if it is safe or forbidden.

MF	Milk Free
DF	Dairy free, includes cheese
CF	Corn Free
WF	Wheat Free
GF	Gluten Free

More on Allergies

There are different types of allergies, for which you can be tested. There are genetic allergies, and there are intolerances, which can also be genetic. The culprits are often corn, wheat, milk protein, dairy or gluten. The tactics in use today to infiltrate our food with gluten, MSG, and corn syrup are sinful. A little knowledge goes a long way toward protecting you and your family.

Some food allergies are brought on by over-exposure to certain foods, and some are brought on by a leaky gut. Check with your practitioner about a cleanse and/or gut reconditioning, which can help immensely.

From what we know at this point in time, a genetic allergy is one you will always have. Any time you consume the allergen, you have put a stressor on your body and a variety of symptoms may manifest. The symptoms may vary, but the following are classic examples:

- Lack of energy
- Joint pain
- Congestion
- Ear ache
- Digestive difficulties
- Skin rashes

NAET —Allergy Elimination

The Nambudriped's Allergy Elimination Technique (known more commonly as NAET) was developed by Devi Nambudriped. This system of allergy elimination works with food, environmental allergies, and others that you may be experiencing; for example, latex, chlorine or other substances that may be aggravating to your system. It can also help lessen the symptoms of genetically inherited allergies, if you are careful to consume the allergen only once in a while. Once a month works for some, once a week for others.

So the rule of thumb would be, for the majority of your diet, you should steer clear of those genetic allergens by using the recipes, or variations thereof, in this guidebook. Only consume the genetic allergen occasionally if you have been through NAET.

Wheat Allergy

Avoid:

Most commercial bread products and pastas, including muffins, pancakes, most rye breads, corn bread, noodles, dumplings, crackers. Semolina, durum, triticale, and graham are types of wheat and also need to be avoided.

- Check all cereals for flour or whole wheat
- Flour tortillas
- Regular soy sauces (Kikkoman, teriyaki, etc.) have wheat
- Suspect all sauces, gravy, thickened soups, stews, and chili
- Foods with any kind of battering or coating. Fried chicken, shrimp, egg rolls, and even some French fries need to be avoided. Many fish and chicken entrees are lightly dusted with flour before cooking.
- Miscellaneous items to check: ice cream, potato chips, corn chips, rice cakes, spices, alcohol (especially beer), extracts with added alcohol, processed meats, sandwich meats and marinades

Substitutes:

- 100% rye bread, millet, amaranth, rice or tapioca bread. Some folks who are wheat allergic can still do spelt, which is an ancient form of wheat. Check with your practitioner. Kamut flour is another substitute.
- Pastas made with spelt, rice, amaranth, corn and quinoa
- Puffed rice, oats, cornmeal, kamut flakes, and buckwheat
- 100% corn tortillas, rice or spelt tortillas
- Wheat-free tamari
- Cornstarch, potato starch, tapioca flour, or a wheat-free flour as a thickener
- Grilled foods are usually wheat free, as are some stir fry entrees

Note: Oats, rye, barley and spelt are often OK, but should be tested for reactivity in people who are wheat allergic because they contain proteins that are similar or identical to those found in wheat.

Corn Allergy

Since we all have different sensitivities, this should be considered a guide rather than a guarantee of corn-free status. This list is always changing as manufacturers are constantly changing their formulas. Watch for any reaction.

Avoid:

Corn

- Corn bread or most multi-grain breads
- Dry cereals — read labels carefully
- Mexican foods — corn chips, taco shells, nachos, corn tortillas
- Popcorn, grits, hominy, masa, hushpuppies
- Corn-on-the-cob, creamed corn, whole-kernel corn

Corn Oil

- Check all baked goods — sometimes called vegetable oil
- Some shortenings (Spectrum non-hydrogenated is OK)
- Sauteed foods
- Non-stick sprays (Pam®)
- Some crackers
- Margarines (any reason to avoid hydrogenated fats is a good one!)

Cornstarch

- Most commercial puddings
- Chinese foods — as a thickener
- Japanese tempura is often cornstarch based
- Some baked products — check baking powder for 'cereal' additives. (Featherweight by Hain group is CF)
- Many cosmetics including baby powder and lipstick
- Salt (cornstarch is sometimes added to reduce caking)

Corn syrup or high-fructose corn syrup

- Soft drinks, many dry cereals, and yogurt
- Most breads, crackers, croutons, cookies (may also be called modified food starch)
- Many pre-made desserts, including ice cream
- Jams, jellies, and peanut butter
- Some salad dressings
- Catsup, pickles, relish, spaghetti sauces and most barbeque sauces
- Chinese sauces — mandarin orange sauce, oyster sauce, duck sauce
- Processed meats, including hot dogs
- Some cheeses, especially Neufchatel

Corn syrup is a cheaper sweetener than many alternatives. Health food stores often will have corn-free varieties but expect to pay a little more. Corn-allergic people have a wonderful opportunity to increase the overall quality of food in their diet by avoiding it.

Substitutes:

See corn-freefoods.blogspot.com for a more complete corn-free/gluten-free list.

FOR	USE
1 teaspoon of baking powder	1/2 teaspoon cream of tartar and 1/4 teaspoon baking soda
Processed meats	Roast your own and slice
Ice cream	Make your own (see our recipe)
Pam cooking spray	Olive oil
Soda	Sparkling water with fresh fruit juices

Milk Allergy

Avoid lactalbumin:

- All milk — skim, lactose free, chocolate, buttermilk, canned, condensed, half-and-half, whey, milk proteins or milk solids
- Yogurt and ice cream

Lactalbumin may be in:

- Gravies, white sauces and cream soups
- Baked goods — watch pancakes, muffins, waffles, breads
- Many desserts — especially cream-based pies, puddings, milk shakes, cakes
- Chocolate (made from milk, corn and cocoa)
- Soft cheeses
- Dried milk (added to many things to increase protein content)
- Deli-meats — especially turkey (for added dried milk)
- Most protein drinks and protein/energy bars
- Cottage cheese, cream cheese, sour cream (Daisy Pure-N-Natural sour cream is OK because there is no milk added to the cream)

Substitute:

- Rice milk, almond milk, oat milk, coconut milk or soy milk
- Goat milk or goat yogurt
- Rice Dream, Tofutti or other non-dairy frozen desserts
- 100% pure cream — can also be mixed with non-dairy drink for a milk-free half-and-half
- Butter is almost always OK for milk reactors

Cheese Allergy*

Avoid casein and lactalbumin:

- All cheese and milk
- Anything with CASEIN in it (ex: sodium caseinate)
- Cheese substitutes — almost all have milk proteins added to them

Substitute:

- Goat, sheep, or buffalo cheese (generally not good for children)
- Rice noodles or corn tortillas — sometimes work in soups or oven dishes
- Added salt — can help offset the lack of cheese

*Look for the DF (dairy free) recipes.

Gluten Allergy

This is not a complete list, so check with manufacturers to verify that an ingredient or food is truly free of gluten.

Some of the following items are also unsafe due to cross-contamination from utensils, equipment, etc., used in their manufacturing.

Abyssinian Hard (Wheat Triticum durum)
Atta Flour (Indian whole wheat flour)
Barley Grass (can contain seeds)
Barley Hordeum vulgare
Barley Malt
Beer — except GF* beer
Bleached Flour
Blue Cheese (made with bread)
Bran
Bread Flour
Brewers Yeast
Brown Flour
Bulgur (Wheat and/or Nuts)
Cereal Binding
Chilton
Club Wheat
Common Wheat
Cookie Dough
Couscous
Criped Rice, or Dinkle (Spelt)
Dextrimaltose
Disodium Wheatgermamido Peg-2 Sulfosuccinate
Durum wheat (Triticum durum)
Edible Coatings
Edible Starch
Einkorn (Triticum monococcum)
Emmer (Triticum dicoccon)
Enriched Bleached Flour

Enriched Wheat Flour
Farina
Farina Graham
Farro
Filler
Flour (normally this is wheat)
Fu (dried wheat gluten)
Germ
Graham Flour
Granary Flour
Groats (barley, wheat)
Hard Wheat
Heeng (Asafoetida)
Hydrolyzed Wheat Gluten
Hydrolyzed Wheat Protein
Hydrolyzed Wheat Starch
Kamut (pasta wheat)
Kluski Pasta
Maida (Indian wheat flour)
Malt
Malted Barley
Malt Extract
Malt Syrup
Malt Flavoring
Malt Vinegar
Macha Wheat (Triticum aestivum)
Matza Semolina
Matzah
Mir
Nishasta (fine starchy powder milled from maize and wheat, used in

Indian puddings and vermicelli)
Oats — except pure oats
Oat Bran — except pure oats
Oat Flour — except pure oats
Oat Groats
Oriental Wheat
Orzo Pasta
Pasta — except those that are GF
Pearl Barley
Persian Wheat
Poulard Wheat
Polish Wheat
Rice Malt (if barley or Koji)
Rolled Oats — except pure oats
Roux
Rye
Seitan
Semolina
Semolina Triticum
Shot Wheat (Triticum aestivum)
Small Spelt
Soy Sauce
Sour Mix — check for exceptions
Spelt (Triticum spelta)
Spirits (check all alcohol)
Sprouted Wheat or Barley
Stearyldimoniumhydroxypropyl
Strong Flour
Suet in Packets

Tabbouleh
Teriyaki Sauce
Textured Vegetable Protein(TVP)
Timopheevi Wheat
Triticale X triticosecale
Triticum Vulgare (wheat — lipids, extract and oil)
Udon (wheat noodles)
Unbleached Flour
Vavilovi Wheat
Vegetable Starch
Vital Wheat Gluten
Wheat, Abyssinian Hard
Wheat Bran Extract
Wheat, Bulgur
Wheat Durum Triticum
Wheat Flour Lipids
Wheat Germ
Wheat Germ Oil
Wheat Grass (can contain seeds)
Wheat Nuts
Wheat Protein
Wheat Triticum aestivum
Wheat Triticum Monococcum
Wheat Bran
Wheat Starch
Whole-Meal Flour
Wild Einkorn
Wild Emmer
Wine Coolers

*GF= gluten free

Use with Caution
(May contain gluten)

Many of the items below can utilize a gluten-containing grain or by-product in the manufacturing process, or as an ingredient. Check with the manufacturer.

Alcohol

Artificial Color

Caramel Color1

(may or may not contain gluten)

Dextrins

Flavoring

Food Coloring

Food Starch

Glucose Syrup

Gravy Cubes

Ground Spices

Maltodextrin

Maltose

Miso

Mixed Tocopherols

Modified Food Starch

Modified Starch

Monosodium Glutamate (MSG)

Mustard Powder

Natural Flavoring

Seasonings

Sirimi

Smoke Flavoring

Soba Noodles

Stabilizers

Starch

Stock Cubes

Suet

Tocopherols

Vegetable Starch

Vegetable Protein

Vegetable Broth

Vitamins

Wheat Starch

(in Europe, the Celiac Society

okays this item)

MSG

To learn more, visit *truthinlabeling.org*. This is the website from which we have pulled information in order to provide you the following list.

HIDDEN SOURCES

OF PROCESSED FREE GLUTAMIC ACID (MSG)

Names of Ingredients That Contain Enough MSG

to Serve as Common MSG-Reaction Triggers

The MSG-reaction is a reaction to free glutamic acid that occurs in food as a consequence of manufacture. MSG-sensitive people do not react to protein (which contains bound glutamic acid) or any of the minute amounts of free glutamic acid that might be found in unadulterated, unfermented food.

These ALWAYS contain MSG

Glutamic Acid	Gelatin
Sodium Caseinate	Textured Protein
Yeast Food	Autolyzed Yeast
Hydrolyzed Corn Gluten	Natrium Glutamate (natrium is Latin/German for sodium)
Monoglycerides	Natural Flavoring

Glutamate

Monosodium Glutamate

Yeast Extract

Hydrolyzed Protein (any protein that is hydrolyzed)

Diglycerides

These OFTEN contain MSG or create MSG during processing

Carageenan   Maltrodextrin
Natural Pork Flavoring   Citric Acid
Bouillon and Broth   Natural Chicken Flavoring
Natural Beef Flavoring   Ultra-pasteurized
Stock   Barley Malt
Whey Protein Concentrate   Pectin
Whey Protein   Protease
Whey Protein Isolate   Protease enzymes
Flavor(s) & Flavoring(s)   Anything Enzyme Modified
Natural Flavor(s) & Flavoring(s)   Enzymes Anything

Malt Extract
Malt Flavoring
Soy Protein Isolate
Soy Sauce
Soy Sauce Extract
Soy Protein
Soy Protein Concentrate
Anything Protein Fortified
Anything Fermented
Seasonings

(the word "seasonings")

In Addition...

The not so new game is to label hydrolyzed proteins as pea protein, whey protein, corn protein, etc. If a pea, for example, were whole, it would be identified as a pea. Calling an ingredient pea <u>protein</u> indicates that the pea has been hydrolyzed, at least in part, and that processed free glutamic acid (MSG) is present. Relatively new to the list are wheat protein and soy protein.

Disodium guanylate and disodium inosinate are expensive food additives that work synergistically with inexpensive MSG. Their use suggests that the product has MSG in it. They would probably not be used as food additives if there were no MSG present.

MSG reactions have been reported to soaps, shampoos, hair conditioners and cosmetics, where MSG is hidden in ingredients that include the words "hydrolyzed," "amino acids," and "protein."

Low fat and no fat milk products often include milk solids that contain MSG. Low fat and no fat versions of ice cream and cheese may not be as obvious as yogurt, milk, cream, cream cheese, cottage cheese, etc., but they are not an exception.

Protein powders contain glutamic, which invariably, would be processed free glutamic acid (MSG). Glutamic acid is not always named on labels of protein powders.

Drinks, candy, and chewing gum are potential sources of hidden MSG, and of aspartame and neotame. Aspartic acid, found in neotame and aspartame (NutraSweet), ordinarily causes MSG type reactions in MSG sensitive people. Aspartame is found in some medications, including children's medications. Neotame is relatively new and we have not yet seen it used widely. Check with your pharmacist.

Binders and fillers for medications, nutrients, supplements, both prescription and non-prescription, enteral feeding materials, and some fluids administered intravenously in hospitals, may contain MSG.

According to the manufacturer, Varivax-Merck chicken pox vaccine (Varicella Virus Live), contains L-monosodium glutamate and hydrolyzed gelatin both of which contain processed free glutamic acid (MSG) which causes brain lesions in young laboratory animals, and causes endocrine disturbances like obesity and reproductive disorders later in life. It would appear that most, if not all, live virus vaccines contain MSG.

Reactions to MSG are dose related, i.e. some people react to even very small amounts. MSG-induced reactions may occur immediately after ingestion or after as much as 48 hours.

Note: There are additional ingredients that appear to cause MSG reactions in ACUTELY sensitive people. A list is available by request from truthinlabeling.org.

Remember: By FDA definition, all MSG is "naturally occurring." "Natural" does not mean "safe." "Natural" only means that the ingredient started out in nature.

Why Pay Attention to the Inflammatory Rating?

- Diabetes
- Excess weight
- Risk of coronary heart disease
- Cancer
- Alzheimers

The Inflammatory Rating estimates the potential of individual foods or combinations of foods to affect the body in a positive or negative way. Hence the positive and negative numbers.

A goal of ours is to create good health, which includes utilizing an abundance of anti-inflammatory foods. Processed sugars and other high-glycemic starches are the enemy.

There is a test you can request from your doctor to measure inflammation. Ask for the "high-sensitivity C-reactive protein," or CRP test.

How to Interpret the Numbers

in the

Nutritional Analysis

In our nutritional analysis at the bottom of each recipe, you will see an inflammatory rating. Foods with positive numbers are considered anti-inflammatory, and those with negative numbers are considered inflammatory. The goal is to make you more aware of your total number for each day. In other words, if you would like to enjoy pancakes some morning, pay attention to the rest of your day, so you can achieve a positive number.

The Top 10 Anti-Inflammatory Foods

1. **Salmon.** *Shopping tip: All salmon from Alaska is wild, whereas Atlantic salmon is usually farmed. Herring, sardines, and tuna also contain omega-3s.*

2. **Grass-fed beef and other animal foods.** Free-range livestock that graze in pastures build up higher levels of omega-3s than grain-fed animals. Slow cooking is helpful with grass-fed beef, as it tends to be a little tougher.

3. **Olive Oil.** Olive oil is a great source of oleic acid, another anti-inflammatory oil.

4. **Ginger.** In addition to it's anti-inflammatory effect, some research suggests that it might also help control blood sugar.

5. **Turmeric.** This spice contains a powerful, natural anti-inflammatory compound.

6. **Cherries.** Eating cherries can significantly reduce inflammation. Cherries are also packed with antioxidants and relatively low on the glycemic index.

7. **Blueberries.** Reduces inflammation and has anti-aging effects for the brain. Eat fresh or frozen.

8. **Salads.** Dark-green lettuce, spinach, tomatoes, and other salad vegetables can help prevent inflammation.

9. **Cruciferous vegetables.** Broccoli, cauliflower, Brussels sprouts, and kale, are all loaded with antioxidants.

10. **Green tea.** A cup a day can also reduce the risk of heart disease, stroke and cancer.

Glycemic Count . . .
and Why it is Important

Glycemic count is a measure of your food's effect on your blood-sugar levels. A normal range would be 100 or less per day. If you are dealing with diabetes or blood-sugar problems, your count should be lower. If you are in good shape and physically active, a little above 100 is acceptable. Consult with your nutritionist or physician to see what is best for you and your dietary goals.

Sodium . . .
and What it Does

Sodium helps to maintain blood volume, regulates the balance of water in the cells, and keeps nerves functioning. Sodium in the form of sea salt, with minerals, and sodium derived from vegetables are helpful for our bodies. Seeing high sodium in some of these recipes, you will want to take this information into account. It is not always the harmful table salt that boosts the sodium count. In vegetables such as beet greens, spinach, carrots and artichokes, the sodium level can be quite high, but in a beneficial manner.

How Many Carbs *do* You Need?

Carbohydrate Formula

The most recent *Dietary Guidelines for Americans* suggests that about half of your daily calories come from carbohydrates. They suggest that a person who eats approximately 2,000 calories per day should take in 250 grams of carbohydrates. This could be why there are so many people developing diabetes and weight problems. For better health, many are striving for 70 grams of carbohydrates per day for weight loss, or due to diabetes. Other health professionals recommend 75 grams per day for maintaining weight and 50-75 grams/day for weight loss. Carbohydrates are sugar and starch, but can be broken down into two categories. It is very important when counting carbs to note which kinds are most prevalent in your diet:

A) Complex Carbohydrates — these are found in grains, vegetables, nuts seeds and legumes.

While keeping track of the amount of carbohydrates you need every day is important, choosing the right carbohydrate-rich foods is equally important. Your main carbohydrate intake should come from fruits and vegetables, and a minor portion from whole grain bread, cereals, pastas, nuts, seeds, and legumes. If focusing on weight loss, stick with fruits, vegetables and some nuts and seeds. Think of no processing, straight from nature!

B) Simple Carbohydrates — these are found in sweet- tasting foods such as flour, sugar, and honey.

Simple carbohydrate-rich foods, such as sugary snacks, pastries, sugar-sweetened soft drinks, candy, cookies, greasy chips and most processed, packaged snack foods should be consumed infrequently or not at all (particularly if you are diabetic). These foods contain too many calories while offering little or no nutritional value. These foods can also contain saturated and trans-fats that are harmful to your health.

Fiber Plays a part

If a bagel has 38 carbohydrates, and 10 grams of fiber, subtract 10 from 38, for a total of 28 grams for your carbohydrate intake.

How Many Calories Do You Need Per day?

You may just want a piece of fruit for a snack, and need the nutritional information to tally in for your day. The most helpful website we've found is *Caloriecountercharts.com* by Mike Vincitorio. It has been given an award by *The Los Angeles Times* recognizing its value to their readership.

Vincitorio includes a modified version of the standard food charts to help you in your weight loss/health journey. He lists most meats, vegetables, fruits, desserts, and dairy. Fiber analysis, however, is not included, and therefore cannot be subtracted from the carbohydrates. Usually, if carbohydrates are listed as 38 grams but there are 10 grams of fiber, then you would only count 28 grams of carbohydrates. So a piece is missing, but nonetheless it is the most useful website we've found to date.

The U.S. Department of Agriculture is the source for all his nutritional information posted in the charts.

Below are examples:

Apples, Raw, Peeled, Sliced   1 Cup
Fat (grams).................................. 0
Food Energy (calories).......... 65
Carbohydrate (grams)............. 16
Protein (grams)......................... .0
Cholesterol (milligrams)............ 0
Weight (grams) 110
Saturated Fat (grams)............. 0.1

Avocados, California   1 Avocado
Fat (grams)...............................29
Food Energy (calories) 322
Carbohydrate (grams) .... .17
Protein (grams) 4
Cholesterol (milligrams) 0
Weight (grams)...................... 201
Saturated Fat (grams) 0.1

Bananas   1 Banana
  Fat (grams) 1
  Food Energy (calories).......... 105
  Carbohydrate (grams) 27
  Protein (grams) 1
  Cholesterol (milligrams) 0
  Weight (grams) 114
  Saturated Fat (grams).............0.2

Beef Steak, Sirloin, Broil, Lean 2.5 Oz.
  Fat (grams)................................. 6
  Food Energy (calories) 150
  Carbohydrate (grams) 0
  Protein (grams) 22
  Cholesterol (milligrams) 64
  Weight (grams)....................... 72
  Saturated Fat (grams) 2.6

Beets, Cooked, Drained, Whole 2 Beets
  Fat (grams) 0
  Food Energy (calories) 30
  Carbohydrate (grams)................7
  Protein (grams) 1
  Cholesterol (milligrams) 0
  Weight (grams)...................... 100
  Saturated Fat (grams) 0

Eggs, Cooked, Poached   1 Egg
  Fat (grams) 5
  Food Energy (calories) 75
  Carbohydrate (grams) 1
  Protein (grams) 6
  Cholesterol (milligrams) 212
  Weight (grams) 50
  Saturated Fat (grams) 1.5

Again, the website for this information is *Caloriecountercharts.com.*

How much protein do you need?

Protein Formula

Body weight x .37 grams is a good standard for daily protein. If working out regularly, your intake can be higher (body weight x 1 gram), and there are many different views for athletes. Some say increase the protein intake while adding more complex carbohydrates. See a nutritional consultant for more specific information.

Another great website for figuring out how much protein you are getting is *www.indoorclimbing.com/Protein_Foods.html*. This site will give you the amount of protein in 3.5 grams of food. It's also a good comparison chart on protein. You may think the 3.5 ounces of steak you ate last night is equal to 3.5 ounces of egg you had in the morning and that the protein content is the same, but it will vary.

The following is an example of their charts which will give you a more exact protein content:

High Protein Foods List:

Animal Protein Foods	1 gram edible protein per 100g (3.5 oz) in weight	Plant and Dairy Protein Foods	1 gram edible protein per 100g (3.5 oz) in weight
Beef Steak, Lean	31.06g	Cheddar Cheese	24.90g
Beef Top Sirloin, Lean	30.55g	Monterrey Cheese	24.48g
Chicken, Dark Meat	28.99g	Almonds	22.09g
Beef Liver	25.51g	Walnuts	15.03g
Cooked Salmon	25.56g	Fried Egg	13.63g

Top 10 Food & Food Ingredients to Avoid

- BHA or BHT
- High fructose corn syrup
- Enriched and bleached flour
- Trans fats and saturated fats
- Artificial colorings
- Fish high in mercury
- Shark, swordfish, tilefish and king mackerel
- Refined sugars
- MSG — monosodium glutamate
- Sodium nitrate
- Artificial sweeteners

These consistently turn up on top 10 lists.

Notes on Roasting

"R" is for roasting. Sweet, essential. No lost nutrients.

I'm going out on a limb here. Everything — meats, vegetables, nuts and mushrooms taste better roasted. There, there, before the howls of protest go up. Hear me out. There are as many good reasons to roast as there are disciples of the venerable and easy way of cooking.

Let's look at easy. At its most basic, roasting involves cooking food in an uncovered pan in an oven. There, that's it. It's a dry-heat method, different from "wet "cooking, like braising, stewing or steaming.

Small pieces of meat, such as tenderloins, roasted at a high heat like 400 °, gain a nicely browned crust with the inside cooked like you like it, and adequately, in a short amount of time. Larger pieces of meat require a low (250 °) to moderate heat (375°). This allows the meat to cook slowly and evenly without burning the outside before it's done.

Veggies also have much to gain by the roasting method. You want to cook them at 395 to 425°. This evaporates their moisture fairly quickly and allows the flavors to concentrate without the veggies burning or over-browning, or becoming too soft. Let's just say it is like attaining the essence of the vegetable. No loss of nutrients either. I have to say here that I strongly suggest roasting vegetables whenever possible. There's usually less to clean up, also.

Yes, there is more. Beets, sweet potatoes, potatoes, and butternut squash all gain from the roasting method, concentrating their natural earth-given sweetness. And if that's not enough, roasting nuts increases the flavor, allowing you to use less in a recipe.

Appetizers

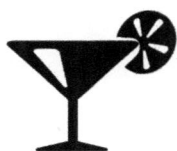

Best Crab Cakes

GF, MF, CF, SF

¾ pound crabmeat
1 cup plain gluten-free
    bread crumbs
¾ cup gluten-free mayonnaise
1 egg, beaten
2 green onions, minced
Hot sauce to taste
Salt and pepper to taste
2 tablespoons olive oil

Serve with the Mango Salsa (p. 101).

Drain the crabmeat. In a large bowl, mix the crabmeat, bread crumbs, mayonnaise, egg, green onions, hot sauce, salt and pepper until combined. Shape the mixture into 16 small cakes. Refrigerate for 30 minutes. Make larger cakes for a main dish.

Heat the olive oil in a large skillet over medium heat. Cook crab cake patties until crisp and golden brown on both sides, about 4 minutes per side. Top with salsa.

Per cake:

Calories	135	Carbohydrates	1.8g
Fat	12g	Fiber	<1g
Cholesterol	16mg	Sugars	0g
Sodium	172mg	Protein	5.18g

Estimated Glycemic Count	1
Inflammatory rating	16.8
Omega-3 fatty acids	828mg

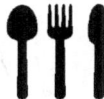

Basic Hummus

GF, DF, CF, SF

The first time we made this, our daughter, Margot, declared it one of the best foods she had ever eaten. From then on, we made it weekly, keeping containers of hummus in the freezer at all times.

2 cups canned garbanzo beans, drained
¼ cup tahini
¼ cup lemon juice
1 teaspoon salt
2 cloves garlic, halved
1 tablespoon olive oil
1 pinch paprika
Fresh parsley, chopped

Place the garbanzo beans, tahini, lemon juice, salt and garlic in a blender or food processor. Blend until smooth. Transfer mixture to a serving bowl.

Drizzle olive oil over the garbanzo bean mixture. Sprinkle with paprika and parsley. Serve warm or cold.

Variations: Add roasted red bell peppers, chopped or blended.

Makes 14 2-ounce servings.

Per Serving			
Calories	189	Carbohydrate	8.5g
Fat	16.8g	Fiber	1.8g
Cholesterol	0mg	Sugars	<1g
Sodium	255mg	Protein	2.26g
	Estimated Glycemic Count	3.2	
	Inflammatory rating	71.4	
	Omega-3 Fatty Acids	131mg	

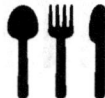

Deviled Eggs

It goes without saying, but we are saying it anyway. Everyone loves deviled eggs. These bright, little treats are perfect for parties, the holidays ,Sunday brunch or most any other occasion.

> 6 eggs, hard boiled
> ¼ cups gluten free mayonnaise *
> ¼ teaspoon dill weed, dried
> ½ teaspoon dry mustard
> Salt and pepper to taste
> Choose from sliced olives, pimentos, shredded carrot, or
>   parsley sprigs for garnish

*Best Foods (Hellmans®) Mayonnaise is GF and SF.

Hard boil six eggs. Once eggs have cooled remove the shells. Cut them in half and remove all the yolks and place on a separate plate. Mash the yolks with a fork.

In a separate bowl mix together the dill weed, dry mustard, gluten free mayonnaise and the mashed yolks. Mix together well. Add salt and pepper to taste.

Take the prepared mixture and spoon it back into the white part of the eggs, and serve.

Serves 6.

Per Serving:			
Calories	146	Carbohydrates	0g
Fat	13g	Fiber	0g
Cholesterol	212mg	Sugars	<1g
Sodium	110mg	Protein	6.3g

Estimated Glycemic Count	<1
Inflammatory rating	-73
Omega-3 fatty acids	534mg

Lima Bean Dip

Fresh, crunchy vegetables and a delicious dip is a great way to get in your daily dose of veggies. This snack/appetizer creates a beautiful presentation due to its verdant color.

> 2 10 oz. packages frozen baby limas, thawed
> One sprig of rosemary
> ½ cup plus 1 tablespoon extra virgin olive oil,
> 2 cloves of garlic, minced
> ¾ cup cured, halved black olives, (reserve some for garnish)
> ¼ cup coarsely chopped flat-leaf parsley
> 2½ tablespoons lemon juice
> Just enough spring-mix greens for presentation on the platter
> 6 sprigs of cilantro
> 2 ounces Romano Pecorino cheese, shaved
> Pink sea salt and freshly ground pepper to taste.

In a large saucepan, heat ¾ cup of the olive oil with the rosemary sprig. Add the thawed lima beans and garlic. Cook over medium heat until the limas are soft, about 10-12 minutes. Drain the beans in a fine sieve set over a heatproof bowl. Discard the rosemary sprig and reserve the oil.

Transfer the lima beans to a food processor and puree. With the machine on, gradually add the reserved oil and process until smooth. Add 2 tablespoons of the lemon juice and season with salt and pepper. Water may be added, a little at time, for a better consistency. This can be made ahead and refrigerated overnight.

In a large bowl, combine the olives, parsley, the remaining 1 tablespoon of oil and ½ tablespoon of lemon juice. Mix in the lima bean puree. Add half of the cheese and toss gently.

Spoon the lima bean puree into a bowl. Place in the center of a platter and surround with a combination of cilantro, a little spring-mix greens, the olives and little shavings of pecorino curled on the top. Serve right away. Pass out the crackers.

Serves 12.

Per Serving for lima bean dip only:

Calories	170	Carbohydrates	11.8g
Fat	11.9g	Fiber	3.5g
Cholesterol	4.8mg	Sugars	<1g
Sodium	216mg	Protein	4.9g

Estimated Glycemic Count	4.2
Inflammatory rating	62.6
Omega-3 Fatty Acids	120mg

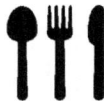

Homemade Corn Chips

GF, DF, SF

Two big pluses for this recipe. It's just too easy, and cuts down calories in a huge way. Compare regular corn chips at 5-7 grams of fat per ounce.

6 corn tortillas

Preheat oven to 400°F.

Take a knife (I like a good pizza cutter) and make 3 equal cross cuts, or imagine a round pizza pie, and you want six slices. You can cut a few tortillas at a time. (Optional: Sprinkle with pink Himalayan salt.

Place these on a baking sheet, and bake for 10-12 minutes, just before they begin to turn brown. I actually like mine slightly brown on the edges.

These are best when served fresh.

Serves 3 (12 chips each).

Per Serving:			
Calories	105	Carbohydrate	21g
Fat	1g	Fiber	3g
Cholesterol	0mg	Sugars	0g
Sodium	22mg	Protein	3g
Estimated Glycemic Count		11	
Inflammatory rating		-79	
Omega-3 fatty acids		16.3mg	

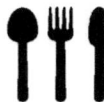

Spinach Crepes

No crepe pan necessary since they're not really crepes.

> 2 teaspoons olive oil
> 1 medium onion, chopped
> 2 cloves garlic, minced
> Bag of pre-washed spinach
> 1 pound of extra lean ground beef
> Salt and pepper to taste
> 2 extra large eggs
> 1 teaspoon coconut oil

In a skillet, warm the olive oil and cook onions until caramelized. Add the garlic, and sauté for two minutes. Add spinach and sauté until soft. Remove from skillet and set aside.

Sauté beef until browned, and drain off any excess fat. Season with salt and pepper, and combine with the onions and spinach.

Place the eggs and coconut oil in food processor or blender.

Cook the egg mixture on a medium griddle as very thin crepes, spread out with the back of a spoon to get it even thinner. Watch for bubbles in center, then flip. The cooked side should be just ever-so slightly brown.

This recipe makes five 5" crepes as a main dish. Small ones are best as they roll up and hold better.

Place 1/5 of spinach/meat mixture on each one and roll up. Serve with sliced tomatoes and a sprig of parsley if a main dish. If using for appetizers, slice the crepes into smaller pieces, and sprinkle the platter with cherry tomatoes and sprigs of parsley. Enjoy!

Serves 5.

Per Serving (1-5" crepe, or cut pieces equaling 1 crepe:			
Calories	253	Fiber	<1g
Fat	12.6g	Sugars	<1g
Cholesterol	162.8mg	Protein	29g
Sodium	328mg		

Estimated Glycemic Count	4.8
Inflammatory rating	5.8
Omega-3 fatty acids	291mg

Rye Parmesan Crackers WF, MF, CF, SF

Quick, hearty snack

Rye crackers (We like Ryvita®)
¼ cup freshly grated Parmesan
Garlic cloves

Rub Ryvita® crackers with a cut clove of garlic. Top each slice with a spoonful of Parmesan and heat through in a toaster oven or under a broiler, being careful to watch closely, until the cheese melts. Serve as an appetizer or with soup.

Per cracker with approximately 1 tablespoon of cheese:

Calories	101	Fat	3g
Fiber	4g	Cholesterol	4.4mg
Sugars	0g	Protein	3.9mg

Estimated Glycemic Count	Info NA
Inflammation Factor	Info NA
Omega-3 Fatty acids	Info NA

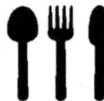

Spinach Crackers

"I love crackers and these are some of the best." Marianne

1 bag of baby spinach
¾ cup almond flour
3 cloves of garlic, minced
2 tablespoons of ghee (or butter or oil)
1 tablespoon water
Salt to taste

Preheat oven to 350°F. In a frying pan melt ghee or butter. Add spinach, garlic, water and salt.

Cover and cook until spinach is wilted and the water is evaporated. Take from the heat and mix in almond flour. Spread on a cookie sheet lined with parchment paper. It should be very thin, about 1/8".

Bake for 25 minutes. Remove from oven and carefully cut into small squares without lifting it from the sheet. Lower the oven to 170°F and bake (dry) for about 60–80 minutes. They are very crispy and hold well together. Although high in calories and (good) fat, these are quite good for glycemics, rate well for anti-inflammatory, low in cholesterol, high in vitamin C and a good source of vitamins A and E.

Calories	94	Carbohydrate	3.4g
Fat	8.25g	Fiber	2g
Cholesterol	3.75mg	Sugars	<1g
Sodium	162mg		

Estimated Glycemic Count   <1
Inflammation Factor   74
Omega-3 Fatty acids   35mg

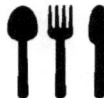

Breakfast

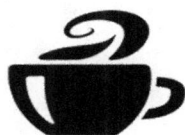

Bran Flax Muffins

My parents took a healthy approach to life. My dad was a jogger in the 50s, and we were introduced to oat bran, wheat germ and other health foods. This is my mother's recipe for bran muffins. They were good then, and they're good now.

2 cups GF flour (p. 177)
¾ cup flaxseed meal
1 cup GF oat bran (Legacy Valley is certified GF)
1 cup brown sugar
2 teaspoons baking soda
1 teaspoon non-aluminum baking powder
2 teaspoons cinnamon
½ teaspoon salt
1½ cup finely shredded or food processed carrots
2 shredded or food processed apples
¾ cup rice or almond milk
2 beaten eggs
1 teaspoon vanilla
½-1 cup chopped nuts (optional)

Mix together first eight ingredients in a large bowl.

Stir in carrots and apples. If adding nuts, do so now.

Combine the liquid with beaten eggs and vanilla. Pour liquid ingredients into dry ingredients. Stir until ingredients are just moistened. DO NOT OVERMIX. Fill muffin cups ¾ full and bake at 350°F for 15 minutes.

Yields 18-21 muffins depending on size of muffin.

Per Serving, 1 muffin			
Calories	151	Carbohydrate	24g
Fat	4g	Fiber	3g
Cholesterol	103mg	Sugars	13g
Sodium	226mg	Protein	6g
Estimated Glycemic Count		13	
Inflammatory rating		NA	
Omega-3 fatty acids		982mg	

Dad's Sunday Morning Spelt & Oatmeal Pancakes

MF, CF

Sunday Morning High Holy Day Treats. Wear your pajamas while eating. They're better that way.

> 1 cup white spelt flour
> 1 cup whole grain spelt flour
> 2 tablespoons aluminum-free baking powder
> ½ cup oatmeal
> 2 tablespoons flaxseeds or flaxseed meal
> 2 eggs
> 3-4 cups low fat soy milk (or almond or coconut milk)
> ¼ cup melted butter or canola oil
> Optional-adding fruit of your choice
> Syrup of your choice

Heat griddle or large skillet or frying pan. Unless you are serving them directly from the griddle, have your oven set to warm for keeping.

Blend dry materials in a large mixing bowl. Whisk wet materials together in a separate bowl and combine with dry materials. Add optional ingredients. Stir well. Small lumps are okay. Don't overmix. Warm the syrup.

Lightly grease the grill, using a pastry brush or a paper towel soaked in oil. Obviously, one needs to be extremely careful with this last method. When griddle is hot enough that a drop of water sizzles, begin cooking pancakes.

Using a ⅓ cup measure as a scoop, pour out as many pancakes as will fit with a little space in between. When the bubbles begin showing through the cakes, flip them. Cook until golden brown, and place on an oven-proof plate so they can keep in a warm oven until ready to serve.

Makes 22-24 5"-pancakes.

Per Pancake:

Calories	81	Carbohydrates	11g
Fat	3g	Fiber	2g
Cholesterol	24mg	Sugar	<1g
Sodium	50mg	Protein	3.5g

Estimated Glycemic Count	6.6
Inflammatory rating	-55

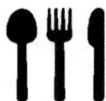

Donnie Cakes Gluten Free

GF, MF, CF

Sunday Morning High Holy Day Treat for those who require gluten free.
We actually prefer these to the regular cakes. You may recognize the following
directions from Dad's Sunday Morning pancakes. Remember, though, gluten-
free cakes take a bit longer to bake solid and they don't bind as well as spelt or
wheat cakes. One must be gentler than one is accustomed to when flipping them.
But they come out great!

2 cups of our GF mix (see p. 177) or pre-made
 GF flour mix.
2 tablespoons aluminum free baking powder
2 eggs
2-3jj cups low fat soy milk (or almond or coconut milk)
¼ cup melted butter or canola oil
Optional to add fruit or nuts: blueberries, bananas,
 strawberries, pecans are all good
Syrup of choice, warmed

Blend dry materials in a large mixing bowl. Separate and whisk the yolks and
whites in separate bowls. Add the yolk mixture first, and blend gently. Then
add the egg white mix. (This step helps gluten-free mixes bind better.)

Add remaining ingredients. Stir well. Small lumps are okay. Don't
overmix.

Lightly grease the grill, using a pastry brush or a paper towel soaked in oil.
Obviously, one needs to be extremely careful with this last method. When
griddle is hot enough that a drop of water sizzles, begin cooking pancakes.
Using a ⅓ cup measure as a scoop, pour out as many pancakes as will fit
with a little space in between. When the bubbles begin showing through
the cakes, flip them (carefully). Cook until golden brown.

Stack on an oven-proof plate and place in a 200° oven to stay warm.

Makes 22-24 5"-pancakes.

Per Pancake:

Calories	109	Carbohydrates	8g
Fat	4g	Fiber	0g
Cholesterol	90mg	Sugars	2g
Sodium	40mg	Protein	4g

Estimated Glycemic Count	1
Inflammatory rating	-40

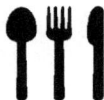

Breakfast for Company

GF, MF, CF, SF

Billye McLaughlin

This was Mom's standard breakfast for large gatherings. Served at the lakehouse and at home, she would easily satisfy 15-20 hungry teenagers with this simple recipe. She used pork, but we're using the leaner turkey in this modified version.

> 1 pound organic turkey sausage
> 6 large eggs, beaten
> 2 small cans of chopped chilis
> ½ pound cheddar cheese, grated

Cook patties of your favorite healthy sausage, and layer a buttered 8½×11" pyrex baking dish with these. This can be done ahead of time, if you prefer. Layer the chopped green chilies, then the grated cheese on top of the sausage. Pour the eggs over it all, and bake at 350°F for about 25 minutes, until eggs hold firm and the top is a nice golden brown.

Serve with some hot biscuits.

Serves 8.

Per Serving:

Calories	319	Carbohydrate	2.8g
Fat	24.5g	Fiber	.5g
Cholesterol	330mg	Sugars	.5g
Sodium	682mg	Protein	221g

Estimated Glycemic Count	1.75
Inflammatory rating	-206
strongly inflammatory	
Omega-3 Fatty Acids	308mg

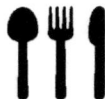

Vegetarian
&
Other Dishes

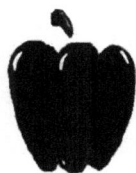

Asparagus with Parmesan

GF, MF, CF, SF

2 pounds asparagus, trimmed
Salt and freshly ground pepper to taste
¼ cup freshly grated Parmesan cheese
1½ tablespoons butter

Steam asparagus until bright green, about 3 minutes. Rinse under cold water. Preheat oven to 425°F.

Butter a 2 quart baking dish and layer the asparagus in rows, with tops covering ends so tips are exposed. Sprinkle each row with cheese and dot with butter.

Bake on upper rack of oven until light crust begins to form and the dish begins to bubble. Remove from oven and serve.

Serves 6 as a side dish.

Per Serving:

Calories	73	Carbohydrates	6g
Fat	4g	Fiber	3g
Cholesterol	11mg	Sugars	3g
Sodium	67mg	Protein	5g

Estimated Glycemic Count   17
Inflammatory rating   83 Mildly anti-inflammatory
Omega-3 fatty acids   34mg

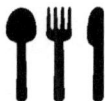

Birthday Polenta

Great when cold outside. In ancient times, polenta was made with chestnut meal. It was originally, and still is, classified as a peasant food.

1 pound sweet Italian turkey sausage
2 pounds boneless chicken breasts or thighs
6 large sage leaves, fresh
2 medium garlic cloves
4 tablespoons rosemary leaves
4 tablespoons olive oil
3 tablespoons unsalted butter
1 cup dry white wine
1 28-ounce can crushed tomatoes
30 large, black, Greek olives, drained
2 cups polenta (ground corn)
4 cups water
2 tablespoons Parmesan, grated
Salt and freshly ground black pepper
¼ cup parsley

Chop the sage, garlic, and rosemary together on a board. Heat the oil and 2 tablespoons butter in a Dutch oven, over medium heat.

When the butter is completely melted, add the chopped herbs and sauté for 2 minutes. Add the sausage and chicken and sauté for 5 minutes, turning them quite often. Add the wine and let it evaporate for 15 minutes.

After the wine is evaporated, add the crushed tomatoes. Season with salt and pepper, cover and cook for 25 minutes.

For the polenta, heat water to boiling. Whisk polenta into water while pouring in a slow stream, stirring continuously until thick and creamy. Stir in the 2 tablespoons of Parmesan and remaining 1 tablespoon of butter.

Chop the parsley and have ready. Add it and the olives to the casserole and mix well. Cook for an additional 10 minutes. Serve immediately over polenta.

Serves 8.

Per Serving:

Calories	349g	Fiber	1.37g
Fat	18g	Sugars	2.75g
Sodium	720g	Protein	36g
Carbohydrates	6.75g		

Estimated Glycemic Count	2
Inflammatory rating	NA

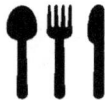

Braised Mustard & Lemon Turnips GF, MF, CF, SF

1 pound turnips
1 tablespoon butter
2 tablespoons Dijon mustard or
   1 tablespoon dry mustard
⅔ cup GF chicken or vegetable broth
2 tablespoons chopped parsley
Juice of half a lemon

Heat the oven to 350°F.

Melt butter in casserole dish in oven.

Pull casserole dish from oven , stir in turnips.

Put back in oven for 7-10 minutes.

Remove and stir in mustard, parsley and broth.

Place back in oven, cook 10-12 minutes.

Remove, add lemon juice, and serve.

These turnips are slightly al dente. If you prefer them to be softer, leave in oven 30-45 minutes.

Serves 4.

Per Serving:			
Calories	77	Carbohydrates	9g
Total Fat	4g	Fiber	2g
Cholesterol	9mg	Sugars	5g
Sodium	219mg	Protein	2g

Estimated Glycemic Count	1
Inflammatory rating	NA
Total Omega- 3 Fatty Acids	96mg

Golden Brussels Sprouts

12 Brussels sprouts
2 teaspoons olive oil
Salt to taste

Wash and cut Brussels sprouts in half. Place face down in skillet with warmed olive oil. Cook covered for about 5 minutes. Uncover and turn up the heat to high for about 3 minutes.

Serves 3.

Per Serving:			
Calories	59	Carbohydrates	6.6g
Fat	3.3g	Fiber	3g
Cholesterol	0mg	Sugars	1.6g
Sodium	794mg	Protein	2.6g
Estimated Glycemic Count		2.6	
Inflammatory rating		69	
Omega-3 Fatty Acids		98mg	

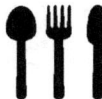

Healthy No-fry French Fries   GF, DF, SF, CF

3 large russet potatoes or 7 small red potatoes
2 tablespoons olive oil
Salt to taste

Preheat the oven to 420°F.

Wash and scrub potatoes thoroughly. Pat dry. Cut the potatoes as you would for thin French fries. Toss thoroughly with the olive oil. Place on an oiled baking sheet, and roast for 30–35 minutes.

Serves 6.

Per Serving:			
Calories	189	Carbohydrates	30g
Fat	4.5g	Fiber	2.3g
Cholesterol	0mg	Sugars	1g
Sodium	10mg	Protein	4g
Estimated Glycemic Count		15	
Inflammatory rating		NA	
Omega-3 fatty acids		70mg	

Satisfy that craving for French fries without all the salt and fat that comes with traditional fries. Spice them up with a little Cayenne.

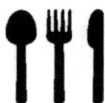

Lettuce Leaf Rollups

GF, DF, CF, SF

2 tomatoes, finely chopped
2 small zucchini, finely sliced
1 teaspoon sweet onion, finely chopped (optional)
1 cucumber, thinly sliced
1 bell pepper, finely diced
1 celery stalk, finely diced
4 large lettuce leaves (butter lettuce works well, or large deep
    green leaves)
1 avocado, peeled and mashed
1 teaspoon fresh lemon juice
Salt and pepper to taste

Mix mashed avocado with lemon juice, herbs. Salt and pepper to taste.
Spread avocado paste on top of large lettuce leaves.

Toss together rest of ingredients and pile on top of avocado. Roll up
leaves, and serve.

Try different vegetables for variation, or add slivered almonds.

Serves 4.

Per Serving:			
Calories:	127	Carbohydrate	14.5g
Fat	8g	Fiber	7g
Cholesterol	0mg	Sugars	6g
Sodium	30mg	Protein	4g
Estimated Glycemic Count		5	
Inflammatory rating		NA	
Omega-3 fatty acids		93mg	

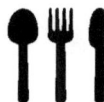

No Wheat Tabouli GF, DF, CF, SF

Forget your wheat allergies by making tabouli with quinoa. Yum!

1 cup quinoa
1 good-sized bunch flat-leaf parsley
1 cup fresh mint leaves (or ¼ cup dried crushed mint leaves)
4 medium tomatoes, peeled, cored, seeded, and chopped
   *(O heresy! You can use a 15-ounce can of diced tomatoes, drained.
   The canned are often more flavorful than the hard balls sold at the
   supermarket these days. Read the label! Canned tomatoes can have
   "natural spices" which can sometimes contain MSG. Of course, use
   homegrown if you have them.*

Dressing:
Juice of 1 lemon (about ¼ cup)
6 green onions chopped (if you don't have green onions,
   chop ⅓ white or yellow onion)
1 clove garlic, crushed
¼ cup extra-virgin olive oil
Salt and freshly ground pepper, to taste

Cover quinoa with 2 cups boiling water, let stand until all water is absorbed.
Fluff with a fork.

Chop the parsley, mint, and garlic (use a food processor if you have one).
Transfer to a small bowl. Add the remaining dressing ingredients, except
the salt, to the bowl and stir to blend. Season with salt to taste and set aside.
Place the quinoa in a medium-size bowl; fluff again. Stir in the dressing and
ingredients; taste for seasoning. Cover and refrigerate for at least 1 hour,
but not more than 4 hours. Adjust the seasoning before serving, adding
lemon juice.

Serves 6.

Per Serving:

Calories	240	Carbohydrates	30g
Fat	11g	Fiber	7g
Cholesterol	0mg	Sugars	2.9g
Sodium	31mg	Protein	7.1g

Estimated Glycemic Count   14
Inflammatory rating   170 strongly anti-inflammatory
Omega-3 fatty acids   322mg

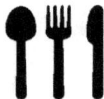

Pepper Flake Broccoli and Cauliflower
(good and simple)   GF, DF, CF, SF

1 pound broccoli heads
½ cauliflower
1 teaspoon red pepper flakes, or to taste
¼ cup rice or other mild vinegar
Salt to taste

Cut broccoli and cauliflower into small flowerets. Cut the broccoli stems into ½-inch slices. Steam all until al dente. Sprinkle with vinegar and red pepper flakes. Salt slightly. Can be served warm or chilled.

Serves 8.

Per Serving:

Calories	26	Carbohydrates	4.8g
Fat	2g	Sugars	1.5g
Cholesterol	0mg	Protein	1.94g
Sodium	20mg		

Estimated Glycemic Count   8.5
Inflammatory rating   217 strongly anti-inflammatory
Omega-3 Fatty Acids   65mg

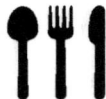

Remarkable Lentils & Rice

GF, MF, CF, SF

Worthy of a potluck offering, take this dish in a crockpot. It makes a great side dish, or main course.

1 cup brown rice, rinsed
½ tablespoon butter
2 cups water
2 cups lentils (green or pink), rinsed*
1 whole onion, medium-large
2 cups GF chicken or vegetable broth
2 carrots, cut into ½" slices
2 tablespoons olive oil
3–4 cups water, depending on desired consistency of lentils
Add more water as needed while cooking
2 tablespoons curry powder, or to taste
1 teaspoon chili powder
Pinch of cumin

Place 1 cup brown rice and 2 cups water in a saucepan. Bring to a boil. Add butter, cover and simmer 40 minutes. In a Dutch oven, or large saucepan, sauté onions and carrots in olive oil until onions are softened. Add seasonings and stir well.

Add lentils, broth, and 1 cup water. Bring to a boil, cover and simmer. Check for any seasonings needed. Add water as needed until desired consistency is reached. Salt and pepper to taste. Stir in rice.

Serves 18.

Pink lentils cook in about 15–20 minutes, green lentils, 1 hour.

Per Serving:			
Calories	54	Carbohydrates	7g
Fat	2g	Fiber	2g
Cholesterol	<1mg	Sugars	1g
Sodium	76mg	Protein	2.7g
Estimated Glycemic Count		3	
Inflammatory rating		NA	
Omega-3 fatty acids		24mg	

Stuffed Tomatoes

GF, MF, CF, SF

Ready in less than an hour, this dish is high in fiber and protein, low in fat. Great summer meal.

4 large tomatoes
1½ cups GF vegetable broth
½ cup sun-dried tomatoes, chopped
1 cup quinoa
6 olives, chopped (green or black)
¼ cup shredded nonfat mozzarella cheese
¼ cup chopped fresh basil
2 tablespoons minced fresh mint leaves
¼ teaspoon ground black pepper

Preheat oven to 375°F (190C).

Cut the fresh tomatoes crosswise in half and scoop out the pulp; set aside. Invert the tomato shells on paper towels to drain.

In a small saucepan, bring the broth and sun-dried tomatoes to a boil. Remove the saucepan from heat and stir in the quinoa. Cover and let stand for 5 minutes.

Stir in the cheese, olives, basil, mint and pepper. Then gently stir in the tomato pulp.

Place the tomato shells in an 11x7-inch baking dish. Spoon the quinoa mixture into the shells, pressing the mixture firmly. Bake at 375°F for 25 to 30 minutes or until heated through.

Serves 4.

Per serving:

Calories	179	Carbohydrates	30.75g
Fat	3g	Fiber	6g
Cholesterol	1mg	Sugars	7.5g
Sodium	267mg	Protein	10g

Estimated Glycemic Count	13
Inflammatory rating	NA
Omega-3 fatty acids	30mg

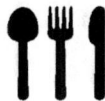

Red Cabbage & Apples

GF, MF, CF, SF

>1 red cabbage, quartered, cored and cut into
>   ¼" slices
>1 teaspoon olive oil
>2 red onions, quartered, then sliced into ¼" slices
>2 apples, washed, peeled & sliced
>½ teaspoon cinnamon
>4 ounces red wine vinegar or red wine
>4 tablespoons water
>1 teaspoon caraway seeds
>2 teaspoons butter to grease the baking dish

Heat the oil in a large pan or wok. Gently sauté the onions, adding in the apples and cinnamon after about 6-7 minutes.

Sauté and stir for 5 minutes longer. Then add the cabbage, caraway seeds, wine (or wine vinegar) and water. Stir well.

Transfer to an ovenproof dish greased with butter. Cover with a tight fitting lid, or foil. Cook for 1-1.5 hours at 375°F.

Variations: Serve with a dollop of goat cheese or dripped yogurt. Garnish with a sprig of parsley.

Serves 6.

Per serving, no cheese or yogurt:			
Calories	118	Carbohydrate	25g
Fat	1g	Fiber	6.8g
Cholesterol	0mg	Sugars	94g
Sodium	163mg	Protein	3.6g
Estimated Glycemic Count		8	
Inflammatory rating		NA	
Omega-3 Fatty Acids		10.8mg	

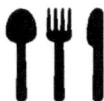

Roasted Beets

GF, DF, CF, SF

2 pounds beets
Kosher salt
Rice (or other mild) vinegar
1 tablespoon olive oil; additional may be necessary

Cut greens from beets and save to have with another meal, or put in covered sauce pan with ¼ cup water or GF broth and cook until wilted.

Preheat oven to 425°F. Chop tops and tails from beets. Toss beets with most of the olive oil, reserving just enough to grease the baking sheet. Roast beets 1 and ½ hour—the more roasted, the sweeter they become, but don't overdo.

Remove from oven and allow to cool. Remove skins and cut into 1-2 inch pieces. Sprinkle with kosher salt and rice vinegar. See Striped Beets and Goat Cheese for a beautiful presentation of this delicious vegetable.

Serves 6.

Per Serving:

Calories	64	Fiber	3.5g
Fat	<1g	Sugars	10g
Cholesterol	0mg	Protein	2.4g
Sodium	504mg		

Estimated Glycemic Count	5
Inflammatory rating	1
Omega-3 fatty acids	7.4mg

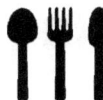

Roasted Vegetables

Our favorite is sweet potatoes, but the following can be used in any combination:

> Onions
> Zucchini or yellow squash
> Bell peppers
> Carrots

Slice about 1/8" thick (¼" for squash and vegetables that cook quickly).

Toss thoroughly with a couple of tablespoons of olive oil.

No nutritional analysis for this, as it will vary depending on the vegetables you use.

It is a standby recipe that we use at least 3-4 times a week.

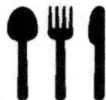

Healthy Butternut Fries

GF, DF, CF, SF

1 tablespoon olive oil
½ butternut squash
Kosher salt

Pre-heat oven to 425°F. Peel and de-seed your butternut squash. If you're unfamiliar with handling them, you may have a little trouble at first. They're fairly easy to peel, but you'll need a sharp knife to cut them. Once your orange friend is peeled and seed-free, slice it in half. Then cut it up into French fry shapes, and toss with most of the olive oil. Reserve a few drops for oiling a cookie sheet.

Place squash on the cookie sheet. Sprinkle lightly with kosher salt (regular salt works, too, but we prefer kosher). Place tray in your pre-heated oven and bake for 40 minutes or so, flipping the pieces halfway through baking process.

Fries are done when they are starting to brown on the edges and get crispy. Serve with ketchup, or however else you enjoy fries or sweet potato fries!

Serving Size: 5 oz., uncooked

Calories	68
Fat	1g
Sodium	486mg
Carbohydrates	16.5g
Fiber	4g
Sugar	3g
Protein	1g

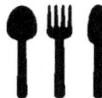

Curry Peanut Casserole

GF, MF, CF, SF

1 large yellow onion
1 medium clove garlic
3-4 medium zucchini
3 medium yellow squash
½ cup sugar-free natural peanut butter
1¼ cups plain nonfat goat yogurt
¼ cup olive oil
¾ cup shredded carrots
1and 1/4 teaspoon curry powder
¼ teaspoon salt
⅛ teaspoon cayenne pepper
1 tablespoon unsalted butter, cut in pieces

Finely chop the onion, mince the garlic and cut the zucchini and yellow squash into 1-inch chunks. Combine the peanut butter and yogurt in a large measuring cup, mixing until it is a uniform tan color.

Position an oven rack in the upper third of the oven; preheat to 400°F. Lightly grease a large shallow casserole dish or gratin dish with nonstick cooking oil spray.

Heat the oil in a large nonstick skillet over medium heat. Add the onion and garlic and cook for 3 to 5 minutes, stirring often, until they have softened. Add the remaining vegetables and cook for 2 minutes, then add the curry powder, salt and cayenne pepper; cook for 1 minute, stirring to mix well. Remove from the heat; add the peanut butter-yogurt mixture and toss to coat evenly.

Transfer to the casserole or gratin dish and dot with the butter. Bake for 20 minutes; the top should be golden brown and the casserole should be bubbling. Some of the vegetables will be crisp-tender. Serve hot.

Serves 10.

Per Serving:

Calories	147	Carbohydrates	11g
Fat	11g	Fiber	3g
Cholesterol	3g	Sugars	4g
Sodium	99mg	Protein	4g

Estimated Glycemic Count   4
Inflammatory rating 68 strongly anti-inflammatory
 Omeg-3 fatty acids   106mg

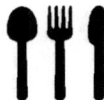

Spicy Coconut Rice with Lime GF, DF, CF, SF

2 cups brown basmati rice
½ of 14-ounce can of coconut milk, lite
1½ cups water
1½ tablespoons olive oil
1 cup minced onions
1 seeded and minced jalapeno pepper
3 teaspoons minced ginger
2 limes, zest and juice (zest is the green part only, not the
white)

In medium saucepan whisk together rice, water and coconut milk. Bring to boil over high, reduce heat, cover, and let simmer 50 minutes. Uncover after 45, and fluff with fork, making sure all liquid is absorbed.

Meanwhile heat oil in sauté pan over medium heat and sauté onions and jalapeno peppers just until translucent and tender. Don't burn. Remove from heat.

Add ginger, onions, jalapeno peppers, lime zest and juice to cooked rice.

Serves 8.

Per Serving:		Sodium	6mg
Calories	209	Carbohydrates	39g
Fat	4g	Fiber	2.4g
Cholesterol	0mg	Sugars	1.58g

Protein	4.28
Estimated Glycemic Count	25.75
Inflammatory rating	125

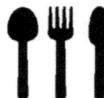

Summer Herbed Potato Salad GF, MF, CF, SF

6 large potatoes, rinsed
1 onion, chopped
½ cup parsley, chopped
1 cup cilantro, chopped
1 teaspoon deli-style mustard
1/3 cup low fat goat yogurt (or low fat mayonnaise)
2 hardboiled eggs chopped
¼ teaspoon cayenne pepper (optional)
Salt and pepper

Boil potatoes until a fork can penetrate the centers. Turn off heat, pour off water and fill the pot with cold water. Leave until potatoes are cold. Drain and peel. Chop potatoes into even-sized cubes and mix gently with onion, parsley and cilantro.

Hardboil the eggs. Cool in iced water. Peel and chop.

In small bowl mix the mustard and mayonnaise. Add to potatoes with chopped eggs. Salt and pepper to taste. Mix gently to combine.

Refrigerate until ready to serve.

Serves 10.

Per Serving:			
Calories:	138	Carbohydrates	19.6g
Fat	4.5g	Fiber	1.9g
Cholesterol	117.1mg	Sugars	2g
Sodium	53.8mg	Protein	5.3g
Estimated Glycemic Count		8.6	
Inflammatory rating		-14.8	
Total Omega-3 fatty acids		151mg	

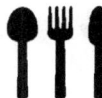

Turnips & Greens

Inexpensive and healthful. Easy and flavorful.

> 2 bunches turnip greens
> 1-2 medium turnips
> 2 tablespoons butter
> 2-3 tablespoons rice vinegar (or to taste)
> Salt and pepper to taste

Peel turnips and chop into small (½-inch) cubes. Place in steamer and begin steaming. While steaming turnips, create a chiffonade, which is rolling the greens and slicing into thin, elegant strips. Add to steamer. Steam everything for 12-15 minutes. Transfer from stove to a pretty bowl, add butter and vinegar, and mix well. Salt and pepper to taste.

You can do the same with beets and their greens. Try steamed chard or the spicy taste of steamed mustard greens. For variation, try lemon juice instead of rice vinegar.

Serves 6.

Per Serving:

Calories	82	Sugars	2.4g
Carbohydrate	8g	Cholesterol	10mg
Fat	4g	Fiber	3g
Sodium	38mg	Protein	1.4g

Estimated Glycemic Count 2
Inflammatory rating 141 strongly anti-inflammatory
Omega-3 fatty acids 85mg

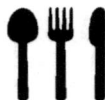

Wild Rice & Carrots

GF, MF, CF, SF

Wild rice is not really rice, but rather a group of grasses grown in low stands of water. It is one of our favorites for its nutty flavor. Wild rice mixed with brown rice or other varieties can be used here. Reduce water if using a variety.

1½ cups wild rice
4½ cups water
3 carrots chopped in ¼" rounds
¼ cup golden seedless raisins
Zest and juice of half an orange
¼ cup parsley
¼ cup pecans
2 tablespoons butter, melted
Salt and pepper to taste

Cook wild rice by bringing water to a boil, then simmering (covered) for 40 minutes. Simmer carrots for 5-7 minutes in a separate saucepan. In a large bowl, mix together all ingredients and serve.

Serves 8.

Per serving:

Calories	140	Carbohydrates	21g
Fat	5g	Fiber	2g
Cholesterol	7mg	Sugars	5g
Sodium	20mg	Protein	3g

Estimated Glycemic Count	9
Inflammatory rating	16
Total Omega-3 fatty acids	106mg

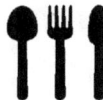

Vegetable Quinoa Medley

GF, MF, CF, SF

If you want to add meat, use chopped chicken, tofu or thin strips of flank steak.

1¾ cups water
1 cup uncooked quinoa
1½ cups small broccoli florets
½ cup finely chopped red onion
⅓ cup shredded carrots
¼ cup raisins
¼ cup dry-roasted cashews, chopped
2 tablespoons white wine vinegar
1½ tablespoons olive oil
1 tablespoon sugar
1½ teaspoons curry powder
2 teaspoons grated fresh ginger
¾ teaspoon salt
1 15-ounce can chickpeas (garbanzo beans), drained and rinsed
¾ cup (3 ounces) crumbled feta cheese

Bring 1¾ cups water to a boil in a medium saucepan; gradually stir in quinoa. Remove from heat; cover and let stand 5 minutes. Fluff with a fork.

While quinoa stands, steam broccoli florets, covered, for 3 minutes or until tender.

In a large bowl, combine quinoa, broccoli, onion, and next 10 ingredients (onion through chickpeas), tossing gently. Sprinkle with cheese.

Serves 6.

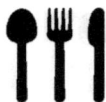

Per Serving:

Calories	408	Carbohydrate	46.8g
Fat	12.2g	Fiber	8.3g
Cholesterol	16mg	Sugars	7g
Sodium	523mg	Protein	15.5g

Estimated Glycemic Count	20
Inflammatory rating	NA
Total Omega-3 fatty acids	192mg

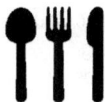

Butternut Squash Rainbow Stew   GF, DF, CF, SF

It's a winner. Presentation and taste.

2 tablespoons butter or olive oil, or one of each
1 large butternut squash, chopped in one-inch chunks
1 large sweet potato, chopped in one-inch chunks
1 onion, chopped
1 bunch mild kale, rolled and cut into thin slices
GF chicken or vegetable broth to cover, at least three cups
1 or 2 large red bell peppers, roasted and peeled
Salt and pepper
¼ cup sherry or vermouth
1 large bay leaf
1 tablespoon wheat-free tamari sauce
1 tablespoon grated fresh ginger (or 1 teaspoon powdered
  ginger)

Put peppers under broiler or on a grill to roast. When charred on all sides, remove, put in plastic bag and refrigerate. (You can do this earlier in the day or buy roasted red peppers in a jar.) This makes it easy to peel the skin off. Also remove ribs and seeds.

Brown onions in Dutch oven about 10 minutes. Stir in chopped squash and sweet potatoes. Heat for another 5 minutes. Add sherry and bay leaf. Let simmer for about 3 minutes. Add broth to cover. If needed add water.

Simmer until squash and potatoes are almost done. Add kale, tamari sauce and ginger, and let cook until kale is done. Add peppers and serve. Pretty and tasty on a cool night.

Serves 6.

Per serving, 356 grams:			
Calories	202	Carbohydrates	32g
Total Fat	7g	Fiber	7g
Cholesterol	10mg	Sugars	8g
Sodium	159mg	Protein	7g
Estimated Glycemic Count		12	
Inflammatory rating		NA	
Omega-3 fatty acids		302mg	

Salads

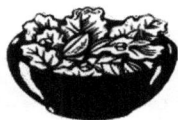

Asian Slaw GF, DF, MF, SF

This can be served as a side dish, or with chicken for a main course.

> 2 cups thinly shredded cabbage (pre-shredded is available in
>   bags in the produce section)
> 1 red bell pepper
> 1 cup fresh bean sprouts
> 1 cup shredded carrots
> ¼ cup Asian peanut dressing (see p. 97)

In a large bowl, toss all ingredients together. Pour in dressing, toss and
serve.

> Optional ingredients:
>   2 cups diced chicken

Serves 2.

Nutritional analysis without sauce or chicken:

Per Serving:			
Calories	63	Carbohydrate	13.5g
Fat	<1g	Fiber	4g
Cholesterol	0mg	Sugars	8g
Sodium	44.5mg	Protein	3g
Estimated Glycemic Count		4.5	
Inflammatory rating		160 strongly anti-inflammatory	
Omega-3 Fatty Acids		30mg	

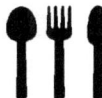

Black Beans and Roasted Corn Salad   GF, DF, SF

This dish is hearty enough to be served as a main meal. Summertime yummy. You have a choice on the corn. A little extra effort on the corn prep can raise this satisfying delight from delicious to nutty tasting and sublime, but is not absolutely necessary.

6 ears of corn, or 2 boxes of frozen corn, or 2 cans of corn
2 15½-ounce cans black beans, rinsed and drained.
1 small red onion, chopped fine
2 avocados, chopped in 1 inch chunks
1 red bell pepper, chopped
1 bunch cilantro, chopped medium
2 jalapenos, seeded and chopped

Dressing:
Juice of one lime
1 teaspoon sugar, agave or honey
2 tablespoons olive oil
Salt and pepper to taste

If using fresh ears of corn (and we hope you do), cut corn from ears. If not, drain or thaw enough to spread corn on oiled cookie sheet and roast for about 7 minutes to enhance the sweetness. Try not to let time constraints that don't allow roasting, or unavailability of corn on the cob, stop you from making this dish. It's a fine dish with canned or frozen corn.

Combine everything, except the avocados and cilantro, which should be added at the last minute.

Make the dressing.

Whisk the lime juice with a couple of tablespoons of olive oil, add the sweetener, and whisk a bit more. At this point, add the avocados and cilantro. Pour dressing over the salad and stir gently.

Note: Cilantro adds a burst of pizzazz at the end, so, depending on your taste for cilantro, you may wish to use a little less of it, but we like the full bunch.

Serves 16.

Per Serving:

Calories	128		
Fat	6g	Sugar	2g
Cholesterol	0mg	Protein	4g
Sodium	11mg	Omega-3 fatty acids	
Carbohydrates	17g	76 mg	
Fiber	5g		
Estimated Glycemic Count		6	
Inflammatory rating		NA	

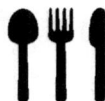

Egg & Tuna Salad Niçoise

3 large eggs
2 tablespoons balsamic vinegar
Sea salt and freshly ground pepper
⅛ cup olive oil
6 cups spring salad mix
2 medium tomatoes, chopped
¼ small red onion, chopped
1 cup artichoke hearts, well drained and sliced
2 6-ounce cans tuna — For no MSG, look for tuna in water,
   no broth. (Whole Foods® is a good brand).
10-12 niçoise or kalamata olives, pitted and chopped
4 medium radishes, thinly sliced

Place the eggs in a saucepan; cover with water. Bring to a boil and cook for 10 minutes. Drain and cool the eggs.

Meanwhile, combine the vinegar, ½ teaspoon salt, and pepper to taste in a small bowl. Whisk in the olive oil. Place the lettuce on each plate, or bowl. Mix the tomatoes, onion and artichokes, olives and radishes.

Divide the tuna evenly among the salads. Peel and thinly slice the hard-boiled eggs and layer the slices over the tuna. Drizzle each with a little of the home-made dressing, or use your own favorite Italian dressing.

Serves 6.

Per Serving:			
Calories	328	Carbohydrates	8.5g
Fat	18g	Fiber	4g
Cholesterol	530mg	Sugars	3.6g
Sodium	451mg	Protein	31.3g
Estimated Glycemic Count		3.3	
Inflammatory rating		7	
Omega-3 fatty acids		331mg	

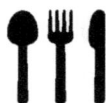

Greek Salad

GF, MF, CF, SF

1 head romaine lettuce — rinsed, dried and chopped
1 red onion, thinly sliced
1 (6 ounce) can pitted black olives
1 green bell pepper, chopped
1 red bell pepper, chopped
2 large tomatoes, chopped
1 cucumber, sliced
1 cup crumbled feta cheese

Dressing:
6 tablespoons olive oil
1 teaspoon dried oregano
1 lemon, juiced
Ground black pepper to taste

In a large salad bowl, combine the romaine, onion, olives, bell peppers, tomatoes, cucumber and cheese.

Whisk together the olive oil, oregano, lemon juice and black pepper. Pour dressing over salad and toss.

Serves 10 side salads, or 5 larger salads.

Per Serving: approximately 2 cups (the smaller salads)			
Calories	106	Carbohydrates	8.4g
Fat	7g	Fiber	3g
Cholesterol	13mg	Sugars	4g
Sodium	322mg	Protein	3.8g
Estimated Glycemic Count		2.8	
Inflammatory rating		NA	
Omega-3 fatty acids		140.8mg	

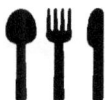

Fattoush

Our beautiful Lebanese neighbor, Rhonda, introduced this, her native dish to us. The coolness of this vegetable dish is a delight in summer.

3 medium firm tomatoes, washed and chopped
3 slender cucumbers, washed and chopped
3 medium radishes, washed and chopped
4 spring onions, washed and coarsely chopped
1 medium onion (¼ cup), roughly chopped
½ cup lemon juice
2 cloves garlic, crushed with a pinch of salt
½ teaspoon dried mint
2 tablespoons vinegar
½ cup olive oil
1 cup coarsely chopped fresh mint leaves
1 cup coarsely chopped parsley
½ cup coarsely chopped sweet green pepper
1 teaspoon salt
8 crisp romaine (2 cups) lettuce leaves, torn into bite-size pieces

For a more authentic version, add ½ teaspoon ground sumac and 1 cup small purslane leaves.

Wash the chopped mint and parsley (and purslane if you are using it). Drain well.

Mix crushed garlic with salt, oil, vinegar, dried mint, lemon juice (and ground sumac if you are using it) and keep aside.

Put all ingredients in a serving bowl and dress with garlic mixture. Mix well.

Serve fattoush garnished with additional toasted GF bread or crackers. Nutritional analysis done without bread.

Serves 10.

Per Serving:

Calories	110	Carbohydrates	12.9g
Fat	6g	Fiber	3.8g
Cholesterol	0mg	Sugars	3.4g
Sodium	281mg	Protein	2.9g

Estimated Glycemic Count	4.5
Inflammatory factor	144 strongly anti-inflammatory
Omega-3 fatty acids	168mg

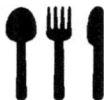

Cranberry Spinach Salad GF, MF, CF, SF

1 tablespoon butter
¾ cup almonds, blanched and slivered
1 pound spinach, rinsed and torn into bite-sized pieces
⅔ cup dried cranberries

Dressing:

2 tablespoons toasted sesame seeds
1 tablespoon poppy seeds
⅛ cup white sugar
2 teaspoons onions, chopped fine
¼ teaspoon paprika
⅛ cup white wine vinegar
⅛ cup cider vinegar
⅛ cup olive oil

In a medium saucepan, melt butter over medium heat. Cook and stir almonds in butter until lightly toasted. Remove from heat, and let cool.

In a large bowl, combine the spinach with the toasted almonds and cranberries.

In a medium bowl, whisk together the sesame seeds, poppy seeds, sugar, onion, paprika, white wine vinegar, cider vinegar, and olive oil. Toss with spinach just before serving.

Serves 8.

Per Serving:

Calories	192	Carbohydrates	16.8g
Fat	13g	Fiber	3.2g
Cholesterol	3.7mg	Sugars	11g
Sodium	39mg	Protein	4.6g

Estimated Glycemic Count 7.3
Inflammatory rating 98 strongly anti-inflammatory
Omega-3 fatty acids 101mg

Spicy Italian Salad

GF, MF, CF, SF

1 bunch broccoli
1 head cauliflower
4 small carrots
Coarse salt
¼ cup sliced black olives

Dressing:
¼ cup olive oil
Juice of 4 lemons
1 teaspoon red pepper flakes

Bring a large pot of water to boiling. Cut the florets from the broccoli and cauliflower. Cut the ends from the broccoli and cauliflower stems. Peel the stems and cut into ½ × 2-inch pieces. Drop in boiling water, or steam for about 5 minutes. Add the florets. Cook for about 4 minutes longer. Meanwhile, scrape the carrots and, using a vegetable peeler, shred them. Put the carrots into a bowl of cold water with ice cubes. Let soak 5 minutes.

Put the oil, lemon juice, and pepper flakes in a glass bowl. Mix together with a wooden spoon (which is best for acidity). Drain the broccoli and cauliflower and put into a serving dish or in a bowl. Pour half the sauce on this and mix well. Drain the carrots and put in bowl. Pour remaining sauce over them. Combine vegetables and mix well.

Serves 12.

Per Serving:			
Calories	81	Carbohydrates	9.2g
Fat	5g	Fiber	3g
Cholesterol	0mg	Sugars	3g
Sodium	50mg	Protein	2.6g
	Estimated Glycemic Count	3.3	
	Inflammatory rating	91	
	Omega-3 fatty acids	62.9mg	

Striped Beets and
Goat Cheese Salad

GF, MF, CF, SF

6 roasted beets (see recipe on page 69)
5 ounces soft goat cheese
½ teaspoon cracked black pepper
6 handfuls of equal parts spring mix and arugula greens

Taking the roasted beets from our recipe on page 69, allow to cool and slice about ¼-inch thick. Mix the goat cheese and pepper together, stirring well.

Place a layer of the goat cheese mix between each slice of beet. Think of frosting between the cake layers. Beets should be the bottom and top (or final) layer. Then holding each beet firmly with one hand, slice each beet into fourths. Place four pieces (one whole beet) on each corner of the salad plate of mixed greens. Stunning.

Serves 6.

Per Serving:			
Calories	128	Carbohydrates	14g
Fat	5.25g	Fiber	4.6g
Cholesterol	10.7mg	Sugars	9.8g
Sodium	203mg	Protein	7g
Estimated Glycemic Count		5.5	
Inflammatory rating	43 strongly anti-inflammatory		
Omega-3 fatty acids		41.5mg	

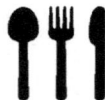

Watermelon and Arugula Salad   GF, MF, CF, SF

1 fresh head of baby arugula, torn into bite-sized pieces
1 half medium red onion, sliced
3 cups seeded watermelon, cubed
¼ cup crumbled feta cheese
10–12 niçoise olives
Fresh oregano

Dressing:
2 teaspoons white wine vinegar
2 tablespoons olive oil
Salt and pepper

Mix together all solid ingredients for salad. For dressing, whisk one part white wine vinegar with 3 parts olive oil. Salt and pepper to taste. Pour on salad, toss and serve.

Note: For a milder salad, use a spring mix instead of the arugula.

Serves 6.

Per Serving:

Calories	95	Carbohydrates	8g
Fat	6g	Fiber	1g
Cholesterol	6mg	Sugars	6g
Sodium	14mg	Protein	2g

Estimated Glycemic Count	2
Inflammatory rating	59
Omega-3 fatty acids	83mg

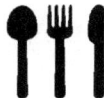

Sauces/Relishes

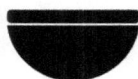

Asian Peanut Sauce

1½ cups creamy peanut butter, reduced fat
½ cup coconut milk, reduced fat
3 tablespoons water
3 tablespoons fresh lime juice
3 tablespoons soy sauce
1 tablespoon fish sauce
1 tablespoon hot sauce
1 tablespoon minced fresh ginger root
3 cloves garlic, minced
¼ cup chopped fresh cilantro

In a bowl, mix the peanut butter, coconut milk, water, lime juice, soy sauce, fish sauce, hot sauce, ginger, and garlic. Mix in the cilantro just before serving. Makes about 24 servings at two tablespoons apiece.

Make the whole recipe, as this sauce can also be served as a dip for vegetables, fondue style or as a dipping sauce for spring rolls. Use what you need and freeze the rest.

Serving size approximately 2 tablespoons:

Per Serving:			
Calories	84	Fats	4.75g
Carbohydrate	5.6g	Cholesterol	0mg
Fiber	<1g	Sodium	259mg
Sugars	1.4g	Protein	4g
Estimated Glycemic Count			2.29
Inflammatory rating			-18

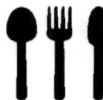

Dr. Bandy's BBQ Sauce

I wrote down the major ingredients while standing in his kitchen. So, this recipe is as close as I can get to the real thing, without him handing me an exact recipe. When he combines this sauce with his 'Green Egg' barbecue pit, it's the best BBQ chicken ever.

It is difficult to find any BBQ sauce that does not have MSG, so beware when eating out.

⅓ –½ cup ketchup (we use HEB/Central Market® for no MSG)

2 tablespoons Paul Newman's Italian Dressing®(GF if you use Light Italian)

1 tablespoon Allegro Marinade®

⅓ cup balsamic vinegar

Juice of 1 lemon

1½ tablespoon mustard, gluten free

1 tablespoon maple syrup

Tabasco® sauce to taste. 2-3 teaspoons makes it mildly hot.

Mix the above ingredients, and either whisk well, or place in a jar with a lid and shake.

Per 1-ounce Serving:

Calories	35	Carbohydrates	6g
Fat	1g	Fiber	0g
Cholesterol	0mg	Sugars	6g
Sodium	212mg	Protein	0g
Estimated Glycemic Count		3	
Inflammatory rating		-18	
Omega-3 fatty acids		52mg	

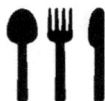

Cranberry Relish

We make it, we have to hide it. If discovered by our daughter, Jamie, it's gone.

1 quart fresh cranberries
4 apples
1 small can crushed pineapple
1 cup agave syrup
1 cup pecans

Grind cranberries in food processor. Remove, then repeat for the apples.

Mix all together and let stand overnight. Taste preferences vary as to the amount of sweetener used. Some may think it bitter without additional sweetening.

Serves approximately 24.

Per 2.6-ounce Serving:

Calories	93	Carbohydrates	17g
Fat	3g	Fiber	2g
Cholesterol	0mg	Sugars	14g
Sodium	14mg	Protein	<1g

Estimated Glycemic Count 7
Inflammatory rating NA

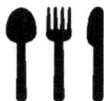

Cranberries and Oranges

GF, DF, CF, SF

No need to limit this one to Thanksgiving or Christmas. And the good news it's moderately anti-inflammatory.

1 quart fresh cranberries
2 6-ounce cans mandarin oranges
1 6-ounce can pineapple
¾ cup agave syrup (or honey)
¾ cup pecans, chopped

Wash and place cranberries in cold water, heat and cook for about 5 minutes. If you see them beginning to burst, remove and drain. Allow to cool and add the other ingredients. Add more agave if needed. Some folks like their relish more on the bitter side, and others on the very sweet.

Serves 10.

Per 3-ounce Serving:

Calories	88	Carbohydrates	9.4g
Fat	5.9g	Fiber	2.6g
Cholesterol	0mg	Sugars	5.6g
Sodium	3.2mg	Protein	1g

Estimated Glycemic Count	1.8
Inflammatory rating	124
Omega-3 Fatty Acids	88mg

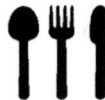

Mango Salsa

Serve this with anything grilled.

1 mango, peeled, pitted and diced
1 red onion, diced
3 tablespoons chopped fresh basil
3 tablespoons chopped fresh cilantro
1 lime, juiced
Minced jalapeno, to taste
Salt and pepper, to taste

In a small bowl combine all ingredients. Refrigerate until ready to use.

Per 1-ounce Serving:

Calories	13	Carbohydrate	3.3g
Fat	<1g	Fiber	<1g
Cholesterol	0mg	Sugars	2.4g
Sodium	2mg	Protein	<1g

Estimated Glycemic Count	1
Inflammatory rating	NA
Omega-3 Fatty acids	5.65mg

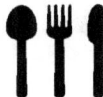

Thai Marinade

Transform your chicken, pork, or tofu into an Asian delight.

1 cup wheat-free tamari sauce
¼ cup rice wine vinegar
1–2 teaspoons chili paste
2 cloves garlic, chopped fine
2 tablespoons grated, fresh ginger root
3 teaspoons toasted sesame oil
1 cup water

Whisk all ingredients together. Use for grilling, broiling or as a stir fry marinade for chicken, pork, or tofu.

Serving size, 4 tablespoons.

Per Serving:			
Calories	57	Carbohydrate	5.26g
Fat	<1g	Fiber	<1g
Cholesterol	0mg	Sugars	<1g
Sodium	368mg	Protein	8.5g
Estimated Glycemic Count		3.2	
Inflammatory rating		88.5	
Omega-3 fatty acid		6mg	

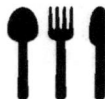

Tomato Spaghetti Sauce

GF, MF, CF, SF
(DF if no Parmesan is used)

Good on chicken, sausage, shrimp, or spaghetti with vegetables. MSG is common in red tomato sauces, so check all cans for wholesome ingredients.

1 16-ounce can petit-dice tomatoes
1 medium onion
3–5 cloves garlic, minced or crushed
¼ cup white wine
1 cup GF chicken broth (MSG alert) or water
Salt to taste
1 tablespoon tomato paste
1 tablespoon dried basil or a small handful of fresh basil
  leaves chopped fine
½ teaspoon powdered thyme
1 tablespoon Thai or Vietnamese fish sauce (optional) or
  four anchovies (optional)
2 tablespoon olive oil
8 ounces gluten-free spaghetti
Water
Freshly grated Parmesan (optional)

Start pot of water for spaghetti.

Heat olive oil in Dutch oven. Sauté onion in oil for 10 minutes or until translucent.

Add garlic. Cook until it starts smelling great.

Add sausage, chicken, or shrimp to onions and garlic, if you want to add protein. Sauté for five minutes or until slightly browned. Add wine, stirring.

Add tomatoes, herbs and broth. Optional are anchovies or fish sauce. Add water to cover. Simmer until meats are done (about 20-30 minutes) while cooking spaghetti in other pot of boiling water.

Drain spaghetti, spoon on sauce and serve. Grate a little fresh Parmesan and add milled pepper if you wish.

Suggested Additions:
Three sweet Italian or Italian herbed sausages (about one pound) chopped into 1½-inch pieces or one pound shrimp. Or one full (both sides) chicken breast (about one pound or more).

This sauce can be served immediately, simmered for an afternoon, or put in the fridge and served the next day.

Serves 8.

Per serving, sauce only:

Calories	64	Carbohydrates	6.1g
Fat	3.8g	Fiber	1g
Cholesterol	<1mg	Sugars	3g
Sodium	17mg	Protein	1.6g

Estimated Glycemic Count	2.5
Inflammatory rating	NA
Omega-3 Fatty Acids	42mg

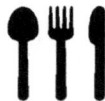

Soups

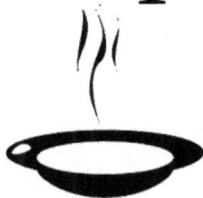

Chicken Mulligan Stew

GF, DF, CF, SF

1 whole chicken
Water to cover
⅓ cup white wine
4 stalks celery, chopped
Salt
3 large carrots, sliced
2 russet potatoes, cubed
1 large onion chopped
2–3 cloves garlic
1 tablespoon olive oil

Cover chicken with water, 1 stalk chopped celery and 1 sliced carrot in large pot. Cover and cook (slow boil) for an hour or until leg bone comes out easily. Save broth to use for stew. Put chicken aside to cool.

Sauté onion in oil until onions are translucent. Add sliced carrots, potatoes, and celery. Sauté for 2 minutes and add wine. Cook for one more minute. Combine all ingredients in the soup pot. Simmer until potatoes are done.

Serves 4.

Per serving:			
Calories	199	Carbohydrates	27g
Fat	6.25g	Fiber	4.5g
Cholesterol	19.25mg	Sugars	6.5g
Sodium	226mg	Protein	8.75g
Estimated Glycemic Count		10.25	
Inflammatory rating		NA	
Omega-3 Fatty Acids		88mg	

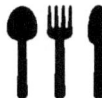

Better-Than-Great Tortilla Soup   GF, MF, SF

There are a couple of steps in here that make this soup rise to the status of "better than great."

> 2 plump boneless chicken breasts, about 1–1½ lbs
> Shredded mild melting cheese, such as Monterrey Jack
> 6 corn tortillas
> 1½ quarts of GF chicken or vegetable broth/water
> 1 quart water
> 1 onion
> 1 15-ounce can diced tomatoes
> 2 small avocados
> 1 cup corn, fresh off the cob
> 1-2 Anaheim peppers
> 2-3 cloves garlic
> 2 teaspoons cumin
> 1½ tablespoons chili powder
> 2 tablespoons olive oil
> Salt and pepper to taste

Greatness step: Make your own corn chips. Preheat oven to 400°F. Cut tortillas into ¾ × 2" strips. Place on baking sheet and salt lightly. Bake at 400°F for about 20 minutes or until the strips turn golden brown. As a substitute, use regular tortilla chips.

Greatness step (optional)—roast corn off cob or frozen corn on cookie sheet while roasting your homemade corn tortilla chips.

Poach the chicken in one quart of the broth. Chop the onion and garlic cloves fine. Stem and seed the peppers (wear gloves if sensitive). Slice peppers into ½"×1½" pieces.

When the chicken is done, remove and let cool. Sauté the vegetables in the oil until soft. Add the seasonings. Put into chicken broth. Meanwhile, for the best results, using two forks shred the chicken or cut into 1-2 inch cubes. Add to the soup. Add the water. Add the tomatoes. Simmer for 20–30 minutes.

Slice avocados thickly. Put two or three slices in bottom of bowl. Add cheese to taste. Pour in hot soup.

Note — if desired, add cooked rice, chopped cilantro, and/or fresh chopped onions. Offer as condiments.

Serves 8.

Per serving:

Calories	316	Total Carbohydrates	18g
Total Fat	16g	Fiber	5g
Cholesterol	61mg	Sugars	2g
Sodium	336mg	Protein	27g

Estimated Glycemic Count	7
Inflammatory rating	NA
Omega 3-fatty acid	168mg

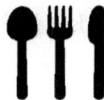

Caldo (A Mexican beef soup)　　　GF, DF, SF

4 cups water
2 cups GF beef broth
¾ pound round steak, sirloin tip or stew meat, trimmed and
　　cut into ½-inch cubes
½ cup salsa
3 garlic cloves, crushed
6 small new potatoes, cut in half
5 carrots, cut in ½" pieces
2 medium onions, cut into large chunks
3 ears of fresh corn, cut into thirds
½ small cabbage, sliced into ¼-inch shreds
1 green pepper, cut into ¾" chunks
1 stalk celery, cut into ½" slices
2 tomatoes, cut into large chunks

Combine water, broth, meat, salsa and garlic in a Dutch oven, or large
stewing pot. Bring to a boil. Reduce heat, cover and simmer 45 minutes.

Add potatoes, carrots and onions. Cover and simmer 15 minutes. Add
remaining vegetables except tomatoes. Cover and simmer 10 minutes. Add
tomatoes and heat through.

To serve, ladle soup into bowls and serve. Top with brown rice if desired.
Drizzle with additional salsa and garnish with lemon, if desired.

Serves 6.

Per serving with no rice and using lean round steak, trimmed:			
Calories	294	Carbohydrates	44g
Fat	4.3g	Fiber	7.9g
Cholesterol	31mg	Sugars	12g
Sodium	485mg	Protein	22.3g
Estimated Glycemic Count		16.8	
Inflammatory rating		204	
Omega-3 Fatty Acids		69mg	

Caldo Made with Chicken

GF, MF, SF, DF

4 cups water

2 cups GF chicken broth (Pacific is a good brand, MSG free)

2 pounds shredded, cooked chicken (if you boil chicken
    first, you can use the broth, then shred)

1 cup salsa

3 garlic cloves, crushed

6 new potatoes, cut in half or bite-sized pieces

5 carrots, peeled and cut in ½" rounds

2 medium onions, processed in food processor

2 cups frozen corn

½ small cabbage, chopped

1 stalk celery, chopped in ½" pieces

1 green pepper, cut into ¾" chunks

2 tomatoes, cut into chunks

Combine liquids, meat, salsa, and garlic in a Dutch oven. Bring to a slow
boil. After about 5 minutes, add potatoes, carrots and onions. Cover and
simmer for 15 minutes.

Add remaining vegetables, except tomatoes. Cover and simmer 10
minutes. Add tomatoes and heat through. Salt and pepper to taste.

Serves 8.

Per Serving:

Calories	264	Sugars	10.5g
Cholesterol	14.5mg	Fat	2.4g
Carbohydrate	51g	Protein	12.8g
Fiber	9g	Sodium	583mg

Estimated Glycemic Count   22
Inflammatory rating   341 strongly anti-inflammatory
Omega-3 fatty acids   157mg

Gazpacho

GF, DF, CF, SF

A recipe shared from our friend, Betty Pearce

1¾ cup tomato juice, from 2 large seeded tomatoes, blended
1¼ cup tomatoes, seeded and chopped
¼ cup onion, minced
1 clove garlic, minced
½ cup red bell pepper, chopped
½ cup green bell pepper, chopped
1 cup cucumber, chopped
¼ cup parlsey, minced
⅛ cup lemon juice
2 tablespoons olive oil
Pinch of sea salt
Dash of black pepper
⅛ cup fresh basil, minced
⅛ cup fresh dill, minced
1 teaspoon celery seed

After blending the 2 large tomatoes, add the remaining ingredients and stir well.

Serves 4.

Per 1 1/4 cup Serving::			
Calories	120	Carbohydrate	13.5g
Fat	7g	Fiber	3.25g
Cholesterol	0mg	Sugars	7.75g
Sodium	17mg	Protein	2.5g
Estimated Glycemic Count		4.25	
Inflammatory rating		NA	
Total Omega-3 fatty acids		70mg	

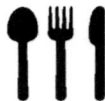

Jalapeno Carrot Soup

2 tablespoons butter
1 medium onion
2 cloves garlic, chopped
2 tablespoons ginger, chopped or grated
½ teaspoon coriander
1 teaspoon cumin
2 pounds carrots, peeled and chopped ½-inch thick
1 jalapeno pepper, seeds removed and chopped
4 cups GF chicken broth (can substitute vegetable broth)
1 cup lite coconut milk
Cilantro, 1/4 cup chopped

In a heavy-bottom pot or Dutch oven, melt butter over medium heat. Add onion, garlic and ginger. Cook until softened but not browned, approximately 3 minutes, stirring frequently.

Stir in coriander and cumin. Add carrots, jalapeno and chicken broth. Simmer covered for 25 minutes, or until carrots are tender.

Transfer soup to blender and blend at high speed until soup is smooth. Pour soup back into pot and add coconut milk. Add salt and pepper to taste.

Serves 4.

Per serving, 2 1/4 cups:			
Calories	251	Sodium	190mg
Fat	14g	Carbohydrates	24g
Cholesterol	12mg	Fiber	6g
		Sugars	10g

Protein	7g
Estimated Glycemic Count	9
Inflammatory rating	NA
Omega-3 fatty acids	45mg

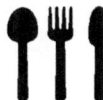

Mushroom Barley Soup MF, CF, SF

This is a comforting winter meal in a bowl based on a classic Central European mushroom and barley soup.

½-ounce dried porcini mushrooms
2 cups boiling water
1 to 2 tablespoons extra virgin olive oil, as needed
1 large onion, chopped
½-pound cremini mushrooms, cleaned, trimmed and sliced thickly
2 large garlic cloves, minced
Salt, preferably kosher, to taste
¾ cup whole or pearl barley
1½ quarts GF chicken broth or water
A bouquet garni made with a few sprigs each thyme and parsley, a bay leaf, and a Parmesan rind
8 to 10 ounces kale, stemmed and washed thoroughly
Freshly ground pepper to taste

Place the dried porcini mushrooms in a bowl or a Pyrex measuring cup, and pour on two cups boiling water. Let sit for 30 minutes. Set a strainer over a bowl, and line it with cheesecloth. Lift the mushrooms from the water and squeeze over the strainer. Then rinse in several changes of water. Squeeze out the water and set aside. Strain the soaking water through a cheesecloth-lined strainer. Add water as necessary to make two cups and set aside.

Heat the oil in a large, heavy soup pot or Dutch oven over medium heat, and add the onion. Cook, stirring often, until just about tender, about five minutes, and add the sliced fresh mushrooms. Cook, stirring, until the mushrooms are beginning to soften, about three minutes, and add the garlic and ½ teaspoon of salt. Continue to cook for about five minutes, until the mixture is juicy and fragrant. Add the reconstituted dried mushrooms, the barley, the mushroom soaking liquid, the bouquet garni and the broth or water. Salt to taste. Bring to a boil, reduce the heat, cover and simmer 45 minutes. Meanwhile, stack the kale leaves in bunches and cut crosswise into slivers.

Add the kale to the simmering soup, and continue to simmer for another 15 to 20 minutes. The barley should be tender and the broth aromatic. The kale should be very tender. Remove the bouquet garni. Season and serve.

Serves 6.

Note: The soup will keep for about three days in the refrigerator, but the barley will swell and absorb liquid, so you may need to add more liquid to the pot when you reheat.

Per 1 1/2 cup Serving:			
Calories	184	Carbohydrate	25g
Fat	5.8g	Fiber	3g
Cholesterol	7mg	Sugars	5.6g
Sodium	350mg	Protein	9.3g
Estimated Glycemic Count		14	
Inflammatory rating		208 strongly anti-inflammatory	
Omega-3 Fatty Acids		130mg	

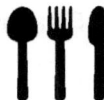

Roasted Tomato Soup

GF, DF, CF, SF

5 tomatoes, cored and quartered
1 red bell pepper, seeded and quartered
3 yellow onions, peeled and quartered
1 tablespoon extra virgin olive oil
5 cloves of garlic, unpeeled
1 teaspoon natural sea salt
2 cups GF vegetable broth
1 cup water
¼ teaspoon paprika

Preheat oven to 375°F. Coat the onion and bell peppers with olive oil. Place all the vegetables on a rimmed baking sheet lined with parchment paper, skin side down. If no paper available, rub the baking sheet with olive oil.

Sprinkle with salt and bake until tomatoes begin to collapse and the onions turn golden. Onions may need turning once to cook more evenly. Cook garlic until golden and soft inside. Peel the garlic.

Place all of the roasted vegetables into a large bowl and puree with a hand blender, or blend in batches in an electric blender or food processor. Add ½ cup of the broth and keep adding ½ cup at a time until the desired consistency is reached. Some like it a little chunky, others smooth. Add the paprika and more salt if needed.

Serves 3.

Per serving:

Calories	134	Carbohydrate	19.6g
Fat	5.3g	Fiber	3.6g
Cholesterol	<1mg	Sugars	7.6g
Sodium	1,049mg	Protein	3g

Estimated Glycemic Count	7.3
Inflammatory rating	500 strongly anti-inflammatory
Omega-3 Fatty Acids	89.3mg

Broccoli Potato Soup   GF, DF, CF, SF

2 tablespoons extra virgin olive oil
1 large onion, chopped
3 garlic cloves, chopped
Salt, preferably kosher, to taste
2 pounds potatoes, peeled and diced
1 bay leaf
2 sprigs each parsley and thyme (optional)
2 quarts water, GF chicken broth, or vegetable broth
1 pound broccoli crowns, coarsely chopped
Freshly ground pepper to taste

Heat the olive oil in a large, heavy soup pot over medium heat and add the onion. Cook, stirring, until tender, about 5 minutes. Add ½ teaspoon salt and the chopped garlic. Cook, stirring, for another minute, until fragrant. Add the potatoes, herbs, water or broth, and salt to taste. Bring to a boil, reduce the heat, cover and simmer 30 minutes. Add the broccoli, turn the heat up slightly to bring back to a boil, then reduce the heat. Simmer uncovered for 10 minutes until the broccoli is thoroughly tender but still bright.

Blend the soup either with a hand blender, or in batches in a blender. Salt, and pepper to taste, and heat through.

Serve with rice or crackers.

Note: The soup can be made hours before serving, or a day ahead, and reheated.

Serves 6–8.

Per Serving:			
Calories	276	Sodium	1246mg
Fat	7g	Fiber	7g
Cholesterol	4mg	Protein	9g
Carbohydrates	45g		

Caudillo

GF, DF, CF, SF

Billye McLaughlin

Marianne writes: When growing up, this soup signaled that fall was here. My mother spent her summers in New Mexico on the Flying B Ranch, a working dude ranch. She was a working cowgirl and her horse, Socks, would fly her way when she whistled. The ranch cook, Ophelia, was rumoured to be a direct descendant of Geronimo, and she taught my mother how to cook caudillo.

> 1 tablespoon olive oil
> 1 pound hamburger meat, lean
> 1 large onion, chopped
> 1 medium potato, peeled and chopped
> 2 carrots, peeled and chopped
> 1 16-ounce can tomatoes
> Water
> 2 tablespoons chili powder, or more to taste
> 2 6 ounce cans of green chiles, or 3-4 fresh, roasted, peeled
>   chiles, chopped
> ½ teaspoon cumin

In a large saucepan, cook onion until clear. Add hamburger, and cook until browned. Add potato, carrots and sauté an additional 5-7 minutes. Add remaining ingredients. Bring to a boil, then simmer covered about 30-40 minutes.

Serves 4.

Per Serving:			
Calories	263	Carbohydrates	23.4g
Fat	6.9g	Fiber	4.5g
Cholesterol	69.5mg	Sugars	7g
Sodium	432mg	Protein	26.7g
Estimated Glycemic Count		7.75	
Inflammatory rating		196	
Omega-3 Fatty Acids		67mg	

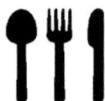

Spinach Sausage Soup

2 pounds sweet organic (turkey or chicken) Italian sausage, casings removed, or organic ground meat, (regular non-organic sausage may be difficult to find without some type of MSG in the seasonings)

2 onions, chopped

4 large carrots, chopped

5 cloves garlic

1 tablespoon olive oil

1.5 quarts GF chicken broth

1.5 quarts water

1 28-oz. can of diced tomatoes (read the label or buy organic to be sure)

1 bunch washed spinach

1 tablespoon dried basil

1/4 cup Parmesan cheese

12 ounce box or bag of small quinoa

Salt and pepper to taste

1 28-oz. can of white or black beans, organic (optional)

While chopping the onion, carrots and garlic, put a pot of water on to boil for the pasta. In a large, heavy soup pot, sauté the onions over medium heat until soft, then add the carrots and garlic. Continue cooking for about two minutes, then add the sausage. Mix well.

Pour in the tomatoes, stir well and heat through. Then add the broth, basil, spinach, and cheese to the soup and simmer, covered, for about 30 minutes.

Gently stir in the cooked pasta, and heat through. (Drained and rinsed beans would be added at this point also, or later individually to each bowl.) Salt and pepper to taste.

Serves 14.

Calories	304	Carbohydrate	29g
Fat	10g	Fiber	5.8g
Cholesterol	44mg	Sugars	4.8g
Sodium	716mg	Protein	25g
Estimated Glycemic Count		13	
Inflammatory rating		169	
Omega-3 fatty acids		200mg	

Simply Incredible Steak Soup GF, DF, CF, SF

2 pounds sirloin or New York strip steak, cut into 2-inch
  squares
1 onion chopped
3 carrots sliced
½ cup frozen peas
½ cup frozen corn
1 bay leaf
2 quarts GF beef broth
1 pint water
2 tablespoons olive oil
1 15 ounce can diced tomatoes
Salt and pepper to taste

Heat oil in Dutch oven. Sauté onion and carrots until the onions are clear, then add the beef and sauté until browned. Add the broth, water and remaining ingredients and simmer until beef is tender—approximately 1½ hours, longer for tougher cuts. Salt and pepper to taste.

Serves 12.

Per Serving:

Calories	202	Carbohydrates	7.9g
Fat	7.5g	Fiber	1.6g
Cholesterol	44mg	Protein	25g
Sodium	526mg		

Inflammatory Rating	50
Estimated Glycemic Count	3.6
Omega-3 fatty acids	38mg

Main Dishes

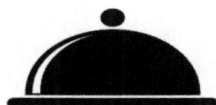

Marinated Red Snapper

2 pounds red snapper fillets (4 medium)
2 tablespoons fresh ginger, minced
1 tablespoon garlic, minced
2 tablespoons olive oil
1 tablespoon fresh lime juice
¼ cup wheat-free tamari sauce
2 tablespoons honey
2 tablespoons dry red wine
⅛ teaspoon cayenne pepper

Whisk all ingredients (except fish) together in glass bowl. Pour over fish, let sit refrigerated for 1–2 hours. Grill, bake, or broil.

Serves 4.

Per Serving:

Calories	331	Carbohydrates	11.25g
Fat	9.7g	Fiber	<1g
Cholesterol	83mg	Sugars	9g
Sodium	941.5mg	Protein	47g

Estimated Glycemic Count	6
Inflammatory rating	NA
Omega-3 fatty acids	908mg

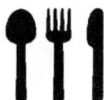

Broiled Tilapia
with Coconut Curry Sauce

GF, DF, CF, SF

Although a little high in fat, the fat from coconut milk is a "good" fat. Coconut milk leaves you very satisfied and full, and is acclaimed to help burn fat.

> 4 6-ounce tilapia fillets
> 1 teaspoon dark sesame oil, divided in half
> 2 teaspoons fresh minced ginger
> 2 cloves garlic
> 1 cup finely chopped green onions
> 1 cup finely chopped red bell peppers
> 1 teaspoon curry powder
> 2 teaspoons red curry paste
> ½ teaspoon ground cumin
> 1 heaping tablespoon brown sugar
> ½ teaspoon salt, divided in half
> ½ of a 14-ounce can of coconut milk, light
> 2 tablespoons fresh cilantro, chopped
> 4 lime wedges

Preheat broiler. Heat ½ teaspoon oil in large skillet over medium heat. Add ginger and garlic. Cool one minute. Add pepper and onions. Cook one minute. Add sugar, ¼ teaspoon salt, curry powder, red curry paste, brown sugar and coconut milk. Bring to a simmer (don't boil). Remove from heat and add cilantro.

Brush fish with ½ teaspoon oil and sprinkle with ¼ teaspoon salt. Place on baking sheet coated with cooking spray. Broil 7 minutes or until fish flakes.

Serve fish on bed of rice, or best on Spicy Coconut Rice with Lime, page 74. Spoon sauce over.

Serves 4.

Per serving:			
Calories	312	Carbohydrates	9.5g
Fat	10.9g	Fiber	2.7g
Cholesterol	95mg	Sugars	6g
Sodium	393mg	Protein	45g
Estimated Glycemic Count		4.75	
Inflammatory rating		149.5	

Tarragon Chicken Rolls

GF, MF, CF, SF

4 chicken breast halves, pounded flat
4 ounces cream cheese (Regular cream cheese is milk free;
    low-fat is not. See p.16 for explanation of milk allergy.)
1 tablespoon tarragon
Almond or brown rice flour for dredging chicken
Salt and pepper
2 tablespoons olive oil
1 tablespoon butter
Round toothpicks
Parsley for garnish

Allow cream cheese to reach room temperature, soft enough to work. Mix with tarragon. Spread mixture evenly on breasts. Roll chicken into tubes and fasten with toothpicks.

Melt butter in olive oil. Dredge rollups in almond or brown rice flour and sauté. The nutritional analysis is done with brown rice flour.

You can do a lower fat version by lightly spraying rollups with olive oil spray and baking at 375°F until done. About 30-40 minutes. Easy, elegant, and, satisfying, but NOT GF.

Serves 4.

Per serving:			
Calories	413	Carbohydrate	17g
Fat	23g	Fiber	1g
Cholesterol	116mg	Sugars	1g
Sodium	160mg	Protein	32g
Estimated Glycemic Count		11	
Inflammatory rating		NA	
Omega-3 fatty acid		214mg	

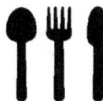

Chicken & Rice
with Carrots & Parsnips

GF, DF, CF, SF

1½ cups. short grain brown rice
2 cups water
1 tablespoon olive oil
1 onion
3 celery stalks, chopped in ¼-inch pieces
5 carrots, cut in bite-sized pieces
2 large parsnips, cut in bite-sized pieces
2 whole chicken breasts
1 cup GF chicken broth
¼ cup white wine
Salt and pepper to taste

Cook the rice separately in a saucepan.

In a large stewing pot, sauté the onion on medium heat until clear.

Add the chicken and sauté until most of the pink is gone, then add the remaining vegetables, stirring frequently for about 5 minutes.

Add the rice, chicken broth, white wine and seasoning. Cover and cook on low heat about 20–25 minutes.

Serves 8.

Per Serving, 203 grams:			
Calories	276	Carbohydrates	39g
Fat	5g	Fiber	4g
Cholesterol	34mg	Sugars	4g
Sodium	121mg	Protein	17.5g
Estimated Glycemic Count		22	
Inflammatory rating		NA	
Omega-3 fatty acids		66mg.	

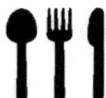

Red Wine Chicken

4 skinless boneless chicken thighs
2 tablespoons olive oil
¼ teaspoon thyme
Pinch salt
¼ cup red wine
Water or GF chicken broth

Wash chicken. Pat dry. Heat oil in 10" heavy skillet.

Season chicken with thyme. Brown on all sides. Turn heat down, pour in wine.

Cook slowly for 40–45 minutes. Add water or broth as needed. When done, place chicken on platter and spoon sauce from skillet over thighs.

Serves 4.

Per Serving:

Calories	132	Carbohydrates	1g
Fat	8g	Fiber	0g
Cholesterol	34mg	Sugars	<1g
Sodium	36mg	Protein	8g

Estimated Glycemic Count	0
Inflammatory rating	NA
Omega-3 fatty acids	92mg

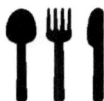

Coconut Curried Chicken & Vegetables

GF, DF, CF, SF

2 tablespoons olive oil

2 pounds chicken, boneless thigh or breast meat, cut into 1-2-inch cubes

¼ cup sherry

1-2 large onion(s), chopped well

1 green bell pepper, chopped roughly—1-2 inches

1 stalk celery, chopped

2 zucchini squash, chopped roughly

1 can lite coconut milk

2 cups GF chicken broth

1 cup water

1 serrano pepper, seeded *(optional, our family likes cuisine a little on the hot side—if no serrano, pepper flakes warm things nicely)*

2 tablespoons Thai fish sauce

2 tablespoons curry powder

1 teaspoon cumin

1 teaspoon chili powder

Juice of one lime (optional)

Using a Dutch oven, brown onion in oil about 10 minutes. Add sherry and scrape onion pieces stuck to pot.

Add the chicken and brown about 5 minutes.

Add vegetables, spices and fish sauce. Mix so that everything is coated with spices.

Add broth to cover. Cook until vegetables are almost done.

Pour in coconut milk. When chicken and veggies are done, add lime juice and serve.

Serves 8.

Per serving:

Calories	281	Carbohydrate	8g
Fat	0g	Fiber	2g
Cholesterol	59mg	Sugars	2g
Sodium	740mg	Protein	30g

Estimated Glycemic Count	3
Inflammatory rating	NA
Omega-3 fatty acids	271mg

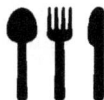

Curried Chicken Legs and Thighs with Mango

(Can be made with both legs and thighs, or either one)

12 pieces chicken (thighs, legs), about 2½ pounds
2 tablespoons butter
Kosher salt
2 tablespoons olive oil
2 large onions, diced (about 4 cups)
6 garlic cloves, chopped
1 4-inch-long piece fresh ginger, peeled and chopped
1 tablespoon garam masala (available in bulk spice section)
1 tablespoon cider vinegar
½ teaspoon cayenne pepper, or more to taste
½ teaspoon ground turmeric
½ teaspoon freshly ground black pepper
⅓ cup unsweetened coconut milk, low fat
2 mangoes sliced into ½-inch cubes (2 cups)
Chopped fresh cilantro or chives for garnish

Trim away fat and skin from sides of chicken pieces, leaving only skin on top. Sprinkle chicken with 1 teaspoon salt.

Heat oil in a large skillet or sauté pan over high heat. Add as many chicken pieces as fit easily, skin side down. Brown chicken on one side, about 6-7 minutes. Turn and brown other side.

While chicken browns, combine 1 cup onion, garlic, ginger, garam masala, vinegar, cayenne, turmeric, black pepper, ½ teaspoon salt and ¼ cup water in a blender, and process until smooth.

Transfer chicken to a glass bowl.

Melt 2 tablespoons butter in skillet over medium heat. Add remaining onions and a large pinch of salt. Sauté until soft, 5 minutes. Add ginger-garlic paste from blender and cook until most of the liquid evaporates, about 2 minutes.

Add coconut milk and 2 cups water, and bring to a simmer. Add mangoes, brown sugar, chicken and any juices that may have accumulated in bowl. Bring to a boil. Cover and turn heat to low, and simmer gently for 1 hour, turning chicken halfway through. Uncover pan, turn chicken again, and let simmer uncovered for 10 minutes.

Spoon any excess fat off sauce and serve garnished with cilantro or chives.

Serves 8.

Per Serving:

Calories	316	Carbohydrate	18g
Fat	14g	Fiber	2.5g
Cholesterol	119mg	Sugars	11g
Sodium	125mg	Protein	29g

Estimated Glycemic Count   5.75
Inflammatory rating   459 strongly anti-inflammatory
Total Omega-3 fatty acids   216mg

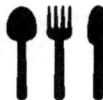

Simple Turkey Chili

GF, DF, CF, SF

- 3 pounds ground turkey
- 1 large onion, chopped
- 2 tablespoons dried garlic granules (2 cloves garlic) or more
- 6 tablespoons San Antonio Chili Powder® or red chili powder
- 2 tablespoons Ancho chili powder
- 1 teaspoon cayenne
- 1 tablespoon cumin
- 1 15-ounce can diced roasted tomatoes with garlic
- 1 small can tomato paste
- ½ cup salsa
- 1 box organic GF chicken or veggie broth
- 2 cups water, add more if needed (sometimes I use wheat-free beer, such as Corona or Dos Equis, instead of water)
- 1 or 2 cans black beans (optional)

Sauté onion in 2–3 tablespoons of broth. Let onions caramelize a bit after broth evaporates.

Add turkey, break up and brown.

Add dry ingredients and mix well.

Add paste, tomatoes, salsa and liquids.

Add beans if desired. Cook on medium heat for at least 30 minutes.

Tips: As the chili cooks, I taste and adjust. The color will tell you if you need to add more chili powder. If you do, use a basic type of powder e.g., New Mexico or just chili powder. (The San Antonio mix has cumin and paprika in it.)

Serves 10.

Per Serving:			
Calories	288	Carbohydrates	12g
Fat	13g	Fiber	3g
Cholesterol	101mg	Sugars	5g
Sodium	604mg	Protein	30g
Estimated Glycemic Count		41	
Inflammatory rating		NA	
Omega-3 fatty acids		218mg	

Down Home Sausage & Rice GF, DF, CF, SF

1 pound of your favorite sausage*, cut into 2-inch pieces
(Low-fat sausages are available at Whole Foods or
specialty markets. Be sure to check for hidden additives;
see MSG list of aliases.)

2 cups brown rice

1 green bell pepper, chopped

2 cups water and 1½ cup GF broth (add more of either later,
if you desire a moister dish)

¼ cup sherry (optional)

1 onion chopped (Your call here, large or small. I think
larger makes the dish sweeter and onions are good for the
blood, so I always add more rather than less.)

1 tablespoon olive oil

In a Dutch oven, sauté onion in oil until soft. Add bell pepper, and stir for
2–3 minutes.

Add sausage and stir occasionally for about 5 minutes. Then add sherry.

Let simmer another 5 minutes, then add rice and 3 cups water or
combination of water and broth. Cover and cook over medium heat for 40
minutes or until rice is done. Cut cooking time in half if you use white rice.
Just remember, if you use white rice, you get little of the nutrition and all of
the simple carbs.

Serves 6.

*MSG free

Per serving:			
Calories	271	Carbohydrate	18g
Fat	12g	Fiber	2g
Cholesterol	69mg	Sugars	<1g
Sodium	561mg	Protein	20g
Estimated Glycemic Count		8	
Inflammatory rating		NA	
Omega-3 fatty acids		267mg	

Greek Turkey Burgers

GF, MF, CF, SF

Flavor up your t-burger!

1 pound ground turkey
1 cup crumbled feta cheese
½ cup green olives, chopped
1 teaspoon dried oregano
1 teaspoon onion powder
½ teaspoon garlic powder
Ground black pepper, to taste

Mix all ingredients together in glass bowl. If you are squeamish about squeezing ground turkey meat with your bare hands, use an electric mixer. Form four patties. Cook as you would hamburgers. You may wish to add a little olive oil to the pan if you are frying, as turkey does not have as much fat as beef and can stick.

Serves 4.

Per Serving:

Calories	182	Sodium	71mg
Fat	12.75g	Carbohydrates	2.5g
Sodium	877mg	Fiber	1g
Cholesterol	81mg	Protein	14.5g

Estimated Glycemic Count   1.5
Inflammatory rating   NA
Total Omega-3 fatty acids   140mg

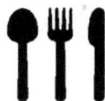

Grilled Moroccan Chicken Breasts   GF, DF, CF, SF

Great with a fresh chopped vegetable salad and a cool, grain salad such as quinoa tabouli!

⅓ cup olive oil (extra virgin)
¼ cup scallions or green onions
⅓ cup chopped parsley
⅓ cup chopped fresh cilantro
1 tablespoon minced garlic
2 teaspoons paprika
2 teaspoons ground cumin
1 teaspoon salt
½ teaspoon turmeric
¼ teaspoon cayenne pepper
4 boneless, skinless chicken breasts, about 2 pounds

Combine oil, scallions, parsley, cilantro, garlic, paprika, cumin, salt, turmeric and cayenne pepper in a food processor or blender.

Process until smooth.

Rub the mixture on both sides of the chicken breasts and let stand 30–60 minutes in fridge.

Grill chicken breasts on medium-hot fire, or broil close to flames 5–7 minutes on each side or until done.

Serves 6.

Per serving, 138 grams:

Calories	305	Carbohydrate	2.16g
Fat	16g	Fiber	<1g
Cholesterol	97.5mg	Sugars	<1g
Sodium	477mg	Protein	36g

Estimated Glycemic Count   <1
Inflammatory rating   502..5 strongly anti-inflammatory
Total Omega-3 fatty acids   178mg

Mole Enchiladas

Okay, so this is not so simple. But imagine having an afternoon in the kitchen making these enchiladas for those you love. Not a recipe after work when you're hurried. Slow down and enjoy the creative process. Involve others. Your family will love you for it!

2 dried ancho chiles (about ¾ ounce)

3 dried mulatto chiles (about ¾ cup)

2 dried pasilla chiles (about ½ ounce) Stores don't always label their chiles, so just select something as close as possible.

2 cups water

2 tablespoons slivered almonds

2 tablespoons unsalted pumpkin seed kernels

1 tablespoon sesame seeds

1 teaspoon olive oil

½ cup chopped onion

2 cloves garlic, crushed

¼ teaspoon ground cinnamon

¼ teaspoon ground cumin

⅛ teaspoon ground cloves

1 (6 inch) corn tortilla, torn into pieces

¾ cup low-salt GF chicken broth (we prefer Pacific)

1 (14½-ounce) can no-salt-added whole tomatoes, drained and chopped

½ teaspoon salt

½ ounce semisweet chocolate, chopped

12 6-inch corn tortillas

3 cups shredded cooked chicken breast (about 1½ pounds skinned and boned chicken breasts)

6 tablespoons (1½ ounces) shredded Monterey jack cheese

Sliced onions, shredded lettuce and sliced radishes (optional)

Remove stems and seeds from chiles. Combine chiles and water in a medium saucepan and bring to a boil; remove from heat. Cover and let stand 1 hour. Drain and set aside.

Combine almonds and pumpkinseed kernels in a small skillet over medium heat. Cook for 5 minutes or until lightly browned, shaking skillet frequently. Remove from skillet, and set aside. Add sesame seeds to skillet, and place over medium heat; cook 2 minutes or until lightly browned, shaking skillet frequently. Remove from skillet and set aside.

Heat one teaspoon olive oil in a skillet over medium heat. Add onion and garlic, and sauté 5 minutes or until tender. Add cinnamon, cumin, and cloves, and cook for one minute, stirring constantly. Set aside.

Place almonds, pumpkinseed kernels, and sesame seeds in a food processor, and process until finely ground. Add tortilla pieces, and process until finely ground. Add chiles, onion mixture, chicken broth, and tomatoes, and process until smooth.

Pour mixture into a medium nonstick skillet. Add salt and chocolate, and cook over low heat 5 minutes or until chocolate melts, stirring frequently. Set the mole aside.

Wrap 12 corn tortillas first in damp paper towels and then in aluminum foil; Alternative method: use tortilla steamer and steam them for about a minute in the microwave until soft and pliable. Spread one tablespoon mole over each tortilla; top each with ¼ cup shredded chicken, and roll up. Place filled tortillas in a 13×9-inch baking dish. Cover and bake at 350°F for 20 minutes.

Arrange 2 enchiladas on each plate; spoon ¼ cup mole over each serving, and sprinkle with 1 tablespoon cheese. Top with sliced onions, shredded lettuce, and sliced radishes, if desired.

Serves 6.

Per Serving:			
Calories	395	Cholesterol	78 mg
Fat	11.5g	Sodium	437 mg
Protein	34.9g		
Carbohydrate	39.9g		
Fiber	5.4g		

Marianne's Chalupas GF, MF, SF

Another family fave and healthier because you make your own tostadas. No frying, no extra calories, or chemicals.

> 1 chicken breast
> ½ cup water
> ½ cup GF chicken broth
> Salt and pepper to taste
> 10 corn tortillas
> 2 16-ounce cans of refried black beans (refried pinto beans, if you like)
> 1 tablespoon olive oil
> 1 teaspoon cumin
> 1 teaspoon chili powder
> 8 ounces lettuce (Romaine is fine, or just use a mix)
> 2 tomatoes, finely chopped
> 1 avocado, sliced
> Handful of cilantro, chopped
> ¾ cup shredded cheddar

Preheat oven to 400°F.

Poach chicken breast in water and broth until just done, with no pink. Allow to cool, then shred.

While chicken is cooking, place 10 corn tortillas on a baking sheet, not overlapping, and bake at 400°F for about 15–20 minutes, or until nice and crispy.

Place 2 cans of refried beans in a saucepan, with the olive oil, cumin and chili powder. Stir until heated through.

Chiffonade the lettuce. This means to roll up a bunch and then make thin slices.

You're ready to assemble your chalupas. Layer in this order:

Beans, chicken, lettuce, tomatoes, cheese, avocado. Enjoy!

Makes 10 chalupas. Serves 5.

Per serving, (2 each):		Sodium	147mg
Calories	530	Carbohydrates	71g
Fat	17g	Fiber	22g
Cholesterol	26mg	Sugars	3g
		Protein	28g

Estimated Glycemic Count	26
Inflammatory rating	NA
Omega-3 fatty acids	388mg

Eggplant Pizza

The eggplant serves as a non-traditional crust, but everyone in our family agrees it's their favorite pizza.

- 1 large eggplant
- 1 pound mozzarella balls (in the cheese section, in containers with water) or you can use shredded mozzarella, pre-packaged
- 1 cup rice flour, white or brown (brown is used in the nutritional analysis)
- 1 onion
- 2 garlic cloves
- 1 teaspoon butter

Additional Pizza Toppings
- 1 large fresh tomato, chopped
- ¼ cup green or black olives, your choice, sliced
- Small handful of fresh basil leaves (dried is fine, but fresh is much better)
- 1 tablespoon of dried oregano. Note: If using fresh, double amount.

Butter the bottom of a pizza pie pan, or an 8×11-inch square pyrex dish.

Wash, but don't peel eggplant. Slice about ¼" thick; dip in water, then into rice flour, both sides. Place the eggplant in the bottom of the dish or pie pan, and overlap as needed. Cook on 400°F for 30 minutes.

Sauté onions until clear, then add garlic. Set aside.

Slice the balls of mozzarella (or open the bag of shredded cheese). Spread this on top of the cooked eggplant. Add tomatoes, olives, cooked onions and any other topping of your choice.

Wash your fresh basil and oregano. Sprinkle on top, and cook for about 15 minutes at 375, or until cheese looks melted.

Serves 6.

Per Serving:

Calories	362	Carbohydrate	30g
Fat	18g	Fiber	5g
Cholesterol	0mg	Sugars	5g
Sodium	534mg	Protein	20g

Estimated Glycemic Count	17
Inflammatory rating	NA
Omega-3 fatty acids	310mg

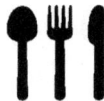

Not Your Mother's Meatloaf GF, DF, CF, SF

2 pounds organic ground beef, the leaner the better (turkey
    can also be used)
1 cup quinoa
1 3/4 cups water
2 onions
1 red bell pepper
½ cup fresh mint or ⅛ cup dried
2 tablespoons fresh basil
½ teaspoon allspice
1 tablespoon cumin
½ teaspoon cinnamon
Salt & freshly ground pepper to taste

Rinse the quinoa, then place in water until soft, cook and drain.

Create a mix of the red bell pepper, onions, mint, basil, allspice, cumin
and cinnamon. Add this mixture to meat and mix all together with cooked
and drained quinoa. Add cool water as needed to soften the mix. Place
combined ingredients in an 8½×11" greased pyrex pan. Bake at 400°F for
30–45 minutes.

Serves 8.

Per Serving:			
Calories	280	Carbohydrate	13g
Fat	14g	Fiber	2.6g
Cholesterol	69.5mg	Sugars	4.75
Sodium	89mg	Protein	24g
Estimated Glycemic Count		4.75	
Inflammatory rating		NA	
Total Omega-3 fatty acids		149mg	

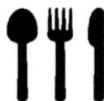

Zesty Orange Grouper

Grouper is a mild fish that is fairly inexpensive.

1½ pounds grouper
1 small orange, peeled and sliced
1 tablespoon lime juice
½ cup chopped onion
2 teaspoons minced garlic
½ tablespoon pepper
1 tablespoon olive oil
1 teaspoon salt

Preheat oven to 350°F.

Cut fish into 4 serving-size pieces and arrange in baking dish.

Combine garlic, lime juice, salt, and pepper. Pour over fish.

Top with chopped onion and place in oven for 12 minutes.

Remove fish from oven, and arrange orange slices over fish.

Cook an additional 5–6 minutes or until fish flakes easily with fork.

Serves 4.

Per serving::

Calories	204	Carbohydrates	5g
Fat	5g	Fiber	1g
Cholesterol	62mg	Sugars	3g
Sodium	380mg	Protein	33g

Estimated Glycemic Count	6
Inflammatory rating	NA
Omega-3 fatty acids	477mg

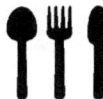

Our Family's Chicken and Dumplings MF, CF, SF
(Noodle dumplings from the South)

This is comfort food at its finest, done with an eye to a lower-fat dish.

4–5 pounds chicken, whole or cut into pieces—or boneless breasts and thighs. *I think using a whole bird makes it more flavorful.*

2 quarts GF chicken broth (we like Pacific Organic low sodium) and/or water

1 large onion, chopped

1 celery stalk, chopped

8–10 sprigs of parsley (optional)

2 carrots, scraped and sliced

1 clove garlic

8 ounces mushrooms, sliced

1 tablespoon olive oil

¼ cup white wine (optional)

Dumplings:

2 cups spelt flour

4 tablespoons butter

2 eggs

First, poach the chicken in enough broth or water to cover. When the chicken is done, let cool, skin, remove from bones, and shred or chop into small chunks. Skim any fat from top of broth. While chicken is cooling, make the dumplings.

Cut the butter into the flour with a pastry cutter or fork until crumbly. Whip the eggs and add all at once to the flour mixture. Mix well until you have a nice ball of dough. Add flour if too wet, or if too dry, add rice milk. Roll to ¼" thick. Slice into 1×2" dumpling pieces.

Heat oil in large pot. Sauté chopped onions for 5 minutes. Add the remaining vegetables, carrots, celery and mushrooms. Sauté for another 5 minutes.

Add the broth and/or water and cooked chicken pieces. Bring to a slow boil.

Add dumpling pieces one at a time. Cook about 5 minutes or until dumplings are cooked.

Serves 12.

Per Serving:

Calories	509	Carbohydrates	32g
Fat	17.5g	Fiber	2g
Cholesterol	185mg	Sugars	3.2g
Sodium	359mg	Protein	52g

Estimated Glycemic Count	21
Inflammatory rating	NA
Omega-3 fatty acids	249mg

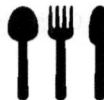

New Mexico Style Red Chili   GF, DF, SF

2 pounds pork loin, cubed (chicken or tofu may be
    substituted, but pork, particularly pork loin, is most
    authentic—pork shoulder can be used also)
2 onions chopped
2 tablespoons olive oil
1 large can posole, drained (a type of corn available on the
    canned vegetable aisle), 36 ounces
4 carrots, peeled and chopped
3 dried Anaheim chiles
2-3 New Mexico red chiles, or good dried chiles
2 teaspoons oregano
2 bay leaves
Salt
Pepper
2 cups water
2 cups GF chicken broth (Pacific is good)

The chiles: don't be daunted by what to do with them. Cover with water and simmer for about 5 minutes or so, until they are reconstituted. Drain most of the water off, remove stems and seeds. Blend with water to make a paste. (Chili powder can be substituted if dried chiles are not available.)

In a large saucepan or Dutch oven, sauté the onions until clear. Add the pork loin and sauté until meat is browned. Add carrots, oregano and bay leaves. Stir a minute, then add water, broth, and stir in chili paste. Simmer until pork is done (tender). Add posole (drained), salt and pepper to taste.

This amazingly soulful dish is the perfect segue into fall.

Serves 10.

Per Serving:			
Calories	322	Carbohydrates	14.9g
Fat	15g	Fiber	2.6g
Cholesterol	83mg	Sugars	2.7g
Sodium	350mg	Protein	26g
Estimated Glycemic Count		5.9	
Inflammatory rating		40	
Omega-3 fatty acids		59mg	

Green Chili Tacos
GF, DF, SF

2 tablespoons olive oil
1 large onion, chopped
2 pounds ground turkey (or ground chicken, or beef)
1 14.5 oz can organic diced tomatoes
2 Hatch chiles roasted & peeled, or can of chiles
2 tablespoons chili
1 teaspoon cumin
Salt & pepper
15 corn tortillas

Cook onions in olive oil in large saucepan until some begin to caramelize. Add turkey and brown. Add spices, then chiles and tomatoes. Heat through.

Wrap in corn tortillas and serve.

Makes about 15 tacos.

Per Taco:			
Calories	176	Carbohydrate	14.6g
Fat	7.73g	Fiber	2.6g
Cholesterol	47.8mg	Sugars	<1g
Sodium	150mg	Protein	12.66g
Estimated Glycemic Count		6.5	
Inflammatory rating		-21 inflammatory	
Total Omega-3 fatty acids		98mg	

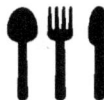

Quick Broiled Fish or Chicken   GF, DF, SF

Use fresh or frozen fish fillets. When you are buying fish, try to buy the wild or wild caught. It has the Omega-3 and Omega-6 balance that makes fish so good for you; 3–6 ounces for each person is about right. This recipe analyzes the orange roughy.

If you prefer chicken, use 6 ounces of chicken thighs per person or 6 ounces of chicken breast each. Use skinless for a lower-fat version.

> Seasonings—salt and pepper. Try different seasonings to change the flavor: thyme, chili pepper, tarragon, paprika, or cayenne for a little kick.

Turn on broiler.

Lightly oil a baking sheet or glass pyrex dish.

Wash fish or chicken and brush lightly with olive oil before seasoning. I suggest doing this to the fish and chicken breasts, particularly if you are going skinless.

Arrange on broiling surface.

Broil the fish and/or breasts about three inches from the heat for about seven minutes on one side, then flip and broil 3 minutes on the other.

With thighs, cook about 10 minutes on one side and three to five on the other.

Quick and easy! Serve with steamed veggies and salad for guilt-free meal.

Per 6-ounce serving of fish:

Calories	129	Carbohydrates	0g
Fat	1.8g	Fiber	0g
Cholesterol	102mg	Protein	27.9g
Sodium	122mg	Sugars	0g

Estimated Glycemic Count	0
Inflammatory rating	102
Omega-3 Fatty acids	39.1mg

Sausage & Sweet Potatoes GF, DF, CF, SF

1 tablespoon olive oil
1 medium onion
3 carrots, chopped in ½-inch pieces
4 celery stalks, chopped
2 sweet potatoes, chopped
3 large links of chicken or turkey sausages
 (If turkey sausage is used, make sure it says natural, organic
 and no MSG.)
Salt and pepper to taste
1 cup brown rice, cooked
1¾ cups water
¾ cup GF chicken broth

Chop sausage into bite-sized pieces and brown in a skillet.

In a large Dutch oven, brown onions until clear, add rest of veggies, and sauté for about 3–5 minutes.

Add cooked sausage, rice, broth and water. Cover with lid and cook about 10–15 minutes.

Serves 8.

Per Serving:			
Calories	339	Carbohydrates	30g
Fat	16g	Fiber	3g
Cholesterol	49mg	Sugars	4g
Sodium	615mg	Protein	17g
Estimated Glycemic Count		16	
Inflammatory rating		NA	
Omega-3 fatty acids		264mg	

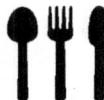

Simple Salmon

2 teaspoons granulated roasted garlic
1 teaspoon salt
1 tablespoon dried basil (optional)
4-6 ounce salmon filets
2 tablespoons butter
4 lemon wedges

Stir together the garlic, basil, and salt in a small bowl; rub equal amounts onto the salmon filets.

Melt the butter in a skillet over medium heat; cook the salmon in the butter until browned and flaky, about 5 minutes per side.

Serve each piece of salmon with a lemon wedge.

Serves 4.

Per Serving:

Calories	294	Carbohydrates	<1g
Fat	16g	Fiber	<1g
Cholesterol	108mg	Sugars	<1g
Sodium	657mg	Protein	34g

Estimated Glycemic Count	<1
Inflammatory rating	803 strongly anti-inflammatory
Omega-3 fatty acids	3461mg

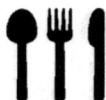

Spicy Burgers

>   1 pound ground turkey, white meat*
>   1 tablespoon olive oil
>   3 tablespoons salsa
>   1 teaspoon Cajun seasoning
>   1 teaspoon salt
>   1 teaspoon (black or white) pepper

Mix all ingredients together in a bowl. Heat olive oil in skillet.
Form four patties and place in skillet when oil is hot. Cook until well done.

Serves 4.

*MSG warning —check your ingredients.

Per Serving:

Calories	199	Carbohydrate	0g
Fat	13g	Fiber	0g
Cholesterol	90mg	Sugars	0g
Sodium	107mg	Protein	20g

Estimated Glycemic Count	0
Inflammatory rating	-62
Omega-3 fatty acids	150mg

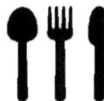

Spiced Braised Beef, Apricots & Chickpeas

GF, DF, CF, SF

This meal has everything you want. It's easy to prep and cook. It's hearty, but not too heavy, richly flavored, multi-textured, fragrant and comforting. Not too bad for a meal that requires only about 15 minutes of prep time.

1½ pounds beef (steak or roast)
2 sweet potatoes—peeled and cut into rounds, then into half moons
1 large sweet onion, chopped
¾ cup chopped dried apricots
1 large (28-ounce) can of whole, peeled tomatoes
2 teaspoons ground cumin
2 teaspoons ground ginger
½ teaspoons ground cinnamon
½ teaspoon cayenne pepper
Sea salt
2 cups cooked quinoa
1 15-ounce can chickpeas/garbanzos, rinsed
3 cups baby spinach, washed well

In a slow-cooker, or 4–6 quart Dutch oven combine the beef, potatoes, tomatoes with their juices, onion, apricots, and spices with ½-cup water.

If using a slow-clooker, cook 4–5 hours on high or 7–8 hours on low. If cooking on stove, cook on low for 4–5 hours.

Twenty minutes prior to serving, cook quinoa. Two cups water to one cup quinoa. Cover and cook on low for 15–20 minutes.

Stir in spinach and garbanzos. Heat through and serve over quinoa.

Serves 8.

Per Serving:

Calories	314	Carbohydrates	42.6g
Fat	5.4g	Fiber	6.9g
Cholesterol	31mg	Sugars	11g
Sodium	393mg	Protein	24.8g

Estimated Glycemic Count	18
Inflammatory rating	NA
Omega-3 fatty acids	44mg

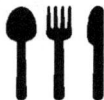

Wild Mushrooms with Chicken Breast

GF, MF, CF, SF

You may find yourself wanting something for a special occasion. You envision a richer sauce than you might normally serve, but you need it to be non-allergic. Buy a heavy cream, with no skim milk added. If you buy the pint of cream, you'll have enough left over to make homemade ice cream for dessert.

¾ cup GF chicken broth
1 ounce dried morels or other wild mushrooms, or a
    combination of two or three
½ pound fresh cultivated mushrooms
4 tablespoons butter, unsalted
¼ cup shallots, finely chopped
⅓ cup port wine
⅓ cup heavy cream
3 chicken breasts, boneless, skinned and halved
Salt and freshly ground pepper to taste
Chopped parsley for garnish

Thoroughly rinse and drain the morels, reserving the liquid. Chop them fine.

Bring the chicken broth to a boil in a small saucepan. Pour it over the wild mushrooms in a small bowl and allow to stand for 2 hours.

Trim stems from the fresh mushrooms and save for another use, or discard. Wipe mushroom caps gently with a damp paper towel and slice thinly.

Melt butter in a skillet, and gently sauté the shallots for 5 minutes, without browning.

Place morels and fresh mushrooms in skillet with salt and pepper and sauté over medium heat for 10 minutes.

Add reserved soaking liquid, the port and heavy cream to the skillet with the mushrooms. Lower heat and simmer for another 5 minutes, or until slightly thickened.

In an 8×11" shallow baking dish, place the mushroom mixture on the bottom. Arrange the chicken breast halves in a single layer on top and cover the dish.

Bake for 20 minutes at 350°F, or until chicken breasts are done. Sprinkle with chopped parsley and serve immediately.

Serves 6.

Excellent with rice and asparagus.

Per serving:			
Calories	161	Carbohydrate	6g
Fat	11g	Fiber	<1g
Cholesterol	50mg	Sugars	1g
Sodium	124mg	Protein	10g
Estimated Glycemic Count		3	
Inflammatory rating		NA	
Omega-3 fatty acids		80mg	

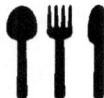

Tilapia & Sweet Potatoes   GF, CF, SF, MF

This different but tasty, and easy-to-make fish recipe makes a great rainy day lunch or main course for dinner. The buttered herbs make a delicious seasoning for sweet potatoes alone.

1½ pounds tilapia filets
3 cups sweet potatoes, peeled and diced small
1 cup salted butter, softened
1 tablespoon fresh cilantro, chopped
1 teaspoon fresh thyme, chopped
1 teaspoon ground allspice
1 tablespoon fresh chives, chopped
½ cup onion, finely chopped
2 teaspoons coarsely ground black pepper
Cilantro sprigs for garnish

Preheat oven to 400°. Grease inside of 9×9"-inch baking pan.

Using a food processor or fork on a plate, blend butter, cilantro, thyme, allspice, chives, onion and black pepper.

Wash fish and pat dry. Place fish inside the baking pan and top with the sweet potatoes. Spread butter-herb combination on top. Cover with lid or aluminum foil.

Bake in the oven for 20 minutes or until sweet potatoes are cooked through. Serve hot garnished with cilantro sprigs and accompanied by a salad. Again, sweet potatoes alone are delicious roasted with the herb butter mix.

Serve 4.

Per Serving:

Calories	340	Carbohydrates	23g
Fat	17.5g	Fiber	4g
Cholesterol	88mg	Sugars	5g
Sodium	108mg	Protein	24g

Estimated Glycemic Count — 9
Inflammatory rating — 183 strongly anti-inflammatory
Omega-3 fatty acids — 264mg

Desserts

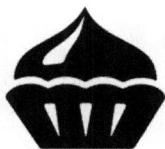

Baked Cinnamon Apples

GF, DF, CF, SF

This is a simple gluten-free dessert, and fairly low in sugar. The idea came from my sister Sheryl, who makes something like this for our parents. Of course, it will not be dairy free or soy free if you add some of the variations below.

> 6 Granny Smith apples, peeled and cut as you would for an apple pie, into about eighths or tenths
> Juice of 1 lemon
> 10 drops of stevia
> 2 tablespoons cinnamon
> ½ teaspoon cardamom
> ⅛ cup agave (or honey)
> ½ cup walnuts or pecans, chopped coarsely

Place the apples in a bowl. Squeeze the juice from the lemon, and add the stevia drops to the lemon juice. Sprinkle over apples. Drizzle with ⅛ cup agave. Toss the apples, coating all surfaces with the lemon juice, stevia and agave. Mix the cinnamon and cardamon, and sprinkle over apples. Add nut pieces, and stir gently. Place apple mixture in an 8½×11" baking dish. Bake at 350°F for 35 minutes.

Variations:

Buy a gluten-free pizza crust and bake with the apples on top.

Serve with our MF ice cream.

Another fun addition is to whisk about 1 and ½ cups warmed soy milk until frothy, then pour over this dessert in small dessert bowls after baking. Sprinkle a little cinnamon on top.

Serves 8.

Per serving (Baked cinnamon apples only):			
Calories	121	Carbohydrates	21g
Fiber	3.3g	Sugars	15.3g
Cholesterol	0mg	Protein	1g
Sodium	<1mg		
Estimated Glycemic Count		5	
Inflammatory rating		-23.6	
Omega-3 Fatty Acids		76mg	

Chickpea Blondies

GF, CF, SF, MF

15 ounces cooked chickpeas, drained and rinsed (also called
  garbanzo beans)
½ cup sugar
½ cup strawberry jam (or other flavor)
¼ cup crunchy peanut butter
2 teaspoons vanilla extract
6 tablespoons flax seed meal
2 tablespoons brown rice flour
½ teaspoon baking powder

Preheat oven to 350°F. Lightly butter an 8"×8"-square baking pan.

In food processor, combine all ingredients and blend until smooth. Scrape
sides often.

Pour batter into pan and bake for 26 minutes.

Cool on wire rack and allow to cool completely before placing in fridge
and slicing.

Serves 16.

Per serving:			
Calories	216	Carbohydrates	24g
Fat	9g	Fiber	4g
Cholesterol	0mg	Sugars	12.3g
Sodium	8mg	Protein	6.9g
Estimated Glycemic Count		11	
Inflammatory rating		NA	

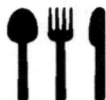

Chocolate Chip Cookies

WF, MF, CF, SF

This recipe originated from sweet Helen Bandy. We have altered it just a bit to reduce fat and sugar content, and it still works beautifully.

¾ cup butter, softened
⅔ cup sugar
⅔ cup packed brown sugar
½ cup peanut butter
1 teaspoon vanilla
2 eggs
2 cups spelt flour, or our GF mix on page 177
1 cup oats
2 teaspoons baking soda
½ teaspoon salt
2 cups chocolate chips, or 1 12-ounce bag (you may substitute carob chips)

Heat oven to 350°F. Mix butter, sugars, peanut butter, vanilla and eggs in large bowl.

Mix in flour, oats, soda and salt. Stir in chocolate chips.

Drop dough by rounded spoonfuls, about 2 inches apart on ungreased cookie sheet. Bake 10–12 minutes or until golden brown. Cool one minute; remove from cookie sheet. Cool on wire rack. Makes about 4 dozen cookies.

Serving size, 2 cookies:

Calories	166	Carbohydrates	21g
Fat	8g	Fiber	2g
Cholesterol	21mg	Sugars	14g
Sodium	186mg	Protein	4g

Estimated Glycemic Count	6
Inflammatory rating	NA
Omega-3 fatty acids	20mg

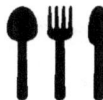

Chocolate Ganache,
or Easy Chocolate Frosting

The easiest way I know to ice a cake with chocolate is to make your own ganache. This recipe can be done in the microwave, or double boiler.

When barely warm, a liquid ganache can be poured over a cake or torte for a smooth and shiny glaze. If cooled to room temperature, it becomes a spreadable filling and frosting.

> 2 tablespoons butter
> ¼ cup soy milk
> 2 teaspoons vanilla (or use cognac or brandy for a different flavor)
> 1 12-ounce bag of chocolate chips (Guittard® is milk free)

This will easily frost an 8×12" sheetcake, or heavily frost an 8×8" 2-layer cake.

Pour the chocolate chips into a glass bowl and microwave on medium, stirring often and watching closely. When they begin to melt, add the butter and soy milk, continuing to heat and stir until all is melted. Stir in the vanilla, and voila! You have an icing that will go between layers of a cake, or wherever needed. While still just warm is the time to pour over your cooled cake.

If there are 12 pieces of cake, each piece will have frosting that will have the following nutritional content:

Per serving:			
Calories	152	Carbohydrates	17.8g
Fat	10g	Fiber	1.6g
Cholesterol	5mg	Sugars	15.4g
Sodium	5.8mg	Protein	1.3g
Estimated Glycemic Count		8	
Inflammatory rating		-87	
Omega-3 fatty acids		26.4mg	

Date Cookies with Coconut GF, MF, CF, SF

Lots of nutritious dates, walnuts and coconut.

½ cup sugar
2 eggs
3 tablespoons butter
½ pound dates, cut up
1½ cups walnuts, chopped
1 cup medium shredded coconut

Preheat oven to 350°F.

Combine the sugar, butter, and eggs in a medium mixing bowl and beat on high speed until light in texture. Stir in the dates, walnuts, and coconut with a wooden spoon.

Grease a cookie sheet with butter or shortening. Drop one teaspoon of batter onto the cookie sheet. Drop another teaspoonful two inches apart from the first one. Repeat until all the batter is gone.

Place pan in center of the oven. Bake 15 minutes or until the coconut is golden in color and the cookies are cooked all the way through. They should only be slightly golden. Let cool on the cookie sheet.

Makes 38 cookies.

Per Serving (One cookie):			
Calories	103	Carbohydrates	10g
Fat	6.9g	Sugars	7g
Cholesterol	13.5mg	Protein	1.5g
Sodium	6.13mg		
	Estimated Glycemic Count	5.4	
	Inflammatory rating	NA	
	Omega-3 Fatty acids	424mg	

Extremely Chocolate Chip Nuggets GF, MF, CF, SF

4 ounces bittersweet chocolate pieces
4 ounces unsweetened chocolate pieces
4 ounces semi-sweet chocolate pieces
6 tablespoons butter
½ cup firmly packed brown sugar
½ cup sugar
3 large eggs
1 tablespoon vanilla extract
⅓ cup rice flour (or spelt if your diet allows)
¼ teaspoon salt
¼ teaspoon baking powder
2 cups very coarsely chopped pecans or walnuts (or both)
12-ounce package MF chocolate chips (Guittard is good.)

Melt chocolates and butter in double boiler, stirring to blend completely. Let cool.

Beat sugars, eggs and vanilla until smooth. Add the melted chocolate and beat until smooth.

Whisk the flour, salt and baking powder together. Add to the chocolate mixture and beat until incorporated.

Stir in nuts and chocolate chips. Let stand 15 minutes.

Drop just a little less than ¼ cup portions onto greased cookie sheet. Bake in 350-degree F oven. Don't overcook these. If the surface starts to crack, you cooked them too long. If you undercook them a little, they stay soft for a week. If you overcook them, they get hard. (The cookies start off dark brown and shiny and change to lighter brown and not so shiny. Then they start to crack.) Don't let them burn on the bottom. Bake 10–15 minutes per sheet, depending on how big you make your cookies.

Makes 36 cookies.

Per cookie:

Calories	182	Carbohydrates	18g
Fat	13g	Fiber	2g
Cholesterol	23mg	Sugars	13g
Sodium	10mg	Protein	3g

Estimated Glycemic Count	9
Inflammatory rating	NA
Omega-3 fatty acids	87mg

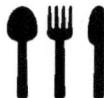

Fruit Crisp

1⅓ cups blueberries (about 6 ounces)
1⅓ cups raspberries
1⅓ cups blackberries
2 large peaches
¾ cup plus 2 tablespoons GF flour
⅓ cup sugar or agave syrup
½ cup light brown sugar
1 teaspoon ground cinnamon
¼ teaspoon ground ginger
Pinch of salt
4 tablespoons unsalted butter, room temperature

Peel, pit and chop the peaches. Butter an 8×8" baking dish and preheat the oven to 350°F.

After rinsing all the berries, toss them with the peaches, agave and 2 tablespoons of the GF flour in a large bowl. Transfer to the buttered baking dish. Bake fruit for 30 minutes, stirring occasionally. Remove from oven.

Meanwhile, whisk remaining ¾ cup GF flour, sugar, cinnamon, ginger and salt in a separate bowl. Cut in butter until evenly distributed. Sprinkle over hot fruit and bake until topping is golden brown, about 20 minutes. It's delicious with our ice cream (p.168).

Serves 8.

Per Serving:			
Calories	213	Carbohydrate	39g
Fat	6g	Fiber	6g
Cholesterol	15mg	Sugars	22g
Sodium	8mg	Protein	3g
	Estimated Glycemic Count	19	
	Inflammatory rating	147	
	Omega-3 fatty acids	94mg	

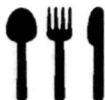

Gayle's Award Winning Cookies   GF, MF, CF, SF

These cookies are GREAT! Simple to make, and impressive to boot. Won "Best Cookie" at an Austin cookie tasting party held by some of the best chefs in town. When I told one of the chefs they were so simple to make, he remarked, "Even better."

> 1 cup light brown sugar
> 1 egg white, beaten until stiff
> 1½ cup chopped pecans, lightly toasted (do not skip toasting)

Toast pecans at 350° for about 10 minutes. Check to be sure that they taste "toasted."

Preheat oven to 400°F. Stir together brown sugar and beaten egg white, and fold in chopped pecans. Drop by heaping tablespoonfuls onto a foil-lined baking sheet.

Turn OFF oven. Place baking sheet in the oven and let them stand for 8 hours. Makes about 4 dozen.

Per Cookie:

Calories	43	Carbohydrate	5g
Fat	2g	Fiber	0g
Cholesterol	0mg	Sugars	5g
Sodium	10mg	Protein	1g

Estimated Glycemic Count	3
Inflammatory rating	NA
Omega-3 fatty acids	34mg

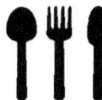

Dairy-Free Ice Cream

GF, DF, CF

A recipe that you can always come up with quickly, if you keep soy milk in the pantry and some frozen fruit in the freezer. There are some great ice cream makers out there now that make this treat quite simple.

> 3 cups plain soy milk (rice dream or almond milk also work, and coconut milk tastes great!))
> ¼ cup honey with about 12 drops stevia (or ¾ cup sugar)
> 1 teaspoon vanilla extract

This makes a great vanilla ice cream. Or the following flavors can be created:
> Blackberry
> Peach
> Coffee
> Chocolate

Place fruit in a blender with ½ cup of the soy. Subtract this amount from the 3 cups required.

If not creamy enough for you, use 1 cup of heavy cream with 2 cups of soy. Be sure the heavy cream is just cream, no skim milk added. Fat and calories go up, but it's a treat, and still MF.

Nutritional analysis is for the vanilla ice cream, with the honey and stevia.

Serves about 6.

Per Serving 1/2 cup for the vanilla with honey and stevia:

Calories	96	Carbohydrates	18g
Fat	1.5g	Fiber	0g
Cholesterol	0mg	Sugars	17g
Sodium	42mg	Protein	2.6g

Estimated Glycemic Count	11
Inflammatory rating	NA
Total Omega-3 fatty acids	0mg

Margot's Muffins

GF, DF, CF, SF

(or known to some as the "Best Banana Oat Bread")

2 tablespoons applesauce
2 tablespoons brown sugar or agave syrup
½ teaspoon vanilla
2 large ripe bananas
½ cup GF flour
1½ teaspoons baking powder
½ teaspoon cinnamon
Pinch of salt
½ cup dry gluten-free oats
Splash of rice milk or almond milk
½ cup walnuts, or other nuts, chopped

Preheat oven to 375. Grease bread or muffin pan. Heat applesauce, brown sugar, and vanilla in a saucepan until it becomes a smooth liquid, and set aside. Peel and mash bananas on a separate plate.

In a separate bowl, sift together flour, baking soda, baking powder, cinnamon, and salt. Then add banana puree and sugar mix from saucepan. Mix together. Add oats and nuts. Add the splash of rice or almond milk.

Pour into pan and cook for about 25-30 minutes or until golden brown on top (15-20 for muffins). Remove and let cool for 5-10 minutes.

Makes 8 slices of bread, or 10 muffins.

Per muffin:			
Calories	125	Carbohydrates	19.7g
Fat	4.6g	Fiber	2.7g
Cholesterol	0mg	Sugars	6.5g
Sodium	2.7mg	Protein	3.4g
Estimated Glycemic Count		9	
Inflammatory rating		-69	
Omeg-3 Fatty acids		549mg	

Pecan-Apple Cake   GF, MF, CF, SF

3 cups peeled, grated apples
3 cups pecan flour (or meal)
⅓ cup melted butter
⅔ cup honey
4 jumbo eggs (or equivalent for smaller ones)
½ teaspoon salt
1 teaspoon baking soda
2 teaspoons cinnamon
1 teaspoon nutmeg
½ teaspoon cloves

Mix apples, pecan flour, butter, and honey.

Beat together eggs, spices, and baking soda.

Blend into pecan flour mix.

Bake in a large, well-buttered pie pan, cake pan, or bundt pan for about 55 minutes at 300°F, or until firm. Or makes 24 muffins.

Per Muffin:

Calories	181	Carbohydrates	11.3g
Fat	15g	Fiber	1.6g
Cholesterol	51mg	Sugars	7.9g
Sodium	115mg	Protein	3g

Estimated Glycemic Count	4.9
Inflammatory rating	-23.79
Omega-3 Fatty Acids	176mg

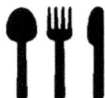

Raspberry Merlot Sorbet

GF, DF, CF, SF

8 ounces frozen raspberries, thawed
1 cup merlot
2 cups water
¾ cup sugar
10 drops stevia
2 tablespoons fresh lemon juice

Mix raspberries and merlot. Puree in blender. Strain to remove the seeds. Heat water to boiling in medium saucepan. Add sugar. Simmer until sugar is completely dissolved. Remove from heat. Add strained raspberry/merlot mixture, stevia and lemon juice. Let cool to room temperature. Chill in refrigerator for one hour. Freeze in ice cream maker about 35 minutes.

Garnish with fresh berries and/or mint leaves (raspberries if available, blueberries are also good.

Serves 6.

Per Serving:

Calories	167.3	Carbohydrates	36g
Fat	0g	Fiber	1.6g
Cholesterol	0mg	Sugars	33.5g
Sodium	1.9mg	Protein	<1g

Estimated Glycemic Count	20.6	
Inflammatory rating	NA	
Omega-3 fatty acids	11mg	

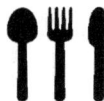

Agave Nut Bars

GF, DF, CF, SF

> 1 cup almond butter (peanut butter can be used)
> 1 cup agave syrup or honey
> 1 cup chopped pecans or almonds
> 1 cup unsweetened coconut
> ¾ cup raw sunflower seeds
> ¼ cup raw sesame seeds
> 1 cup dried cranberries or cherries

Preheat oven to 350°F.

Heat honey and almond butter in a saucepan until melted and smooth.

In a bowl, mix together the pecans, coconut, sunflower seeds, and cranberries or cherries.

Add the melted mixture to the dry ingredients and mix until well combined. Pour into a 9x13-inch casserole dish and press flat.

Bake 20–30 minutes (20 minutes is usually good).

Remove from oven and let cool before cutting into squares.

Store in an airtight container for a great snack.

Approximately 24 servings.

Per Serving:			
Calories	240	Carbohydrate	21.7g
Fat	17.5g	Fiber	3g
Cholesterol	0mg	Sugars	15.5g
Sodium	4.8mg	Protein	3.6g
Estimated Glycemic Count			9.2
Inflammatory rating			-83
Omega-3 fatty acids			102mg

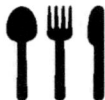

Sugarplums

GF, DF, CF, SF

A favorite of mine for Christmas, or anytime. Can be made one month in advance.

> 2 cups whole almonds... you can buy toasted and save on time
> ¼ cup agave syrup (or honey)
> 2 teaspoons grated orange zest
> 1 ½ teaspoons ground cinnamon
> ½ teaspoon ground allspice
> ½ teaspoon ground nutmeg
> 4-5 tablespoons unsweetened cocoa, depending on your preference (analysis is done with 4)
> 1 cup dried figs, finely chopped
> 1 cup pitted dates, finely chopped
> Confectioners sugar

Preheat oven to 350°F. Arrange almonds on a baking sheet in a single layer and toast in oven for 6-8 minutes. Remove and allow to cool.

Meanwhile, combine honey, orange zest, cinnamon, allspice, and nutmeg in a large bowl. Once cooled, finely chop the almonds. Add almonds, figs, and dates to the spice mix in the large bowl. Mix well with a wooden spoon or your hands. Hands work best, as this mix tends to clump and stick to utensils.

Pinch off rounded teaspoon-sized pieces and roll into balls. Dust with powdered sugar and refrigerate in single layers between sheets of wax paper in airtight containers for up to one month. It seems the longer they sit, the more the flavors come out. Makes approximately 20-25 "plums," depending on size.

Per serving (for 25):

Calories	133	Carbohydrate	20g
Fat	6g	Fiber	3.4g
Cholesterol	0mg	Sugars	15g
Sodium	1.5mg	Protein	3g
Estimated Glycemic Count		9	
Inflammatory rating		NA	
Omega-3 fatty acids		NA	

Gluten-Free
Solutions

Gluten-Free Mix

We make a gluten-free flour by combining rice, potato, and
tapioca flours in a ratio of:

5½ cups rice flour
1 cup potato flour
1 cup tapioca flour

*While there is an abundance of gluten-free flours, such as sweet potato
flour, garbanzo flour, millet, almond flour or meal, soya flour, etc., the above
combination works well.*

For more specific needs, see www.ellenskitchen.com/faqs/glutfree.html.

FYI — tapioca also adds a sweet flavor and makes crispy crusts.

Per 3/4 cup:

Calories	593	Carbohydrates	133g
Fat	2g	Fiber	0g
Cholesterol	0mg	Sugars	0g
Sodium	0mg	Protein	9g

Estimated Glycemic Count 84
Inflammatory rating NA
Omega-3 fatty acids 414mg

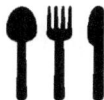

Gluten-Free Websites and All Stars

1. The Essential Gluten-Free Blog
2. *Celiac-disease.com*
3. *Gluten-FreeMall.com*
4. *GFlinks.com*
5. *Glutenfree.com*
6. *LivingWithout.com* (magazine for people who are living gluten free)

Recipes

1. *http://www.triumphdining.com/blog/gluten-free-flour-a-guide*
2. *BeFreeForMe.com* (input your allergies and category e.g., dessert, and it will bring up recipes that work for you. Incredible!

All-Star Products

Pamela's — great baking mix

Pizza crust — Gluten Free Naturals has a mix. Very good.

KinniKinnick — great donuts

Best Gluten free bread

Food for Life — bread — Almond Rice® is best, we also like the millet

Amy's has some gluten-free frozen meals

Ener-G — perfect pretzels

Tasty Snacks

Blue Diamond Nut Crackers® (check for milk)

Energy bars from thinkproducts

Sources

Bandy D.C., John, austinholistichealth.com, March 2009

www.Truthinlabeling.ORG. Jack Samuels. April 2010

www.Caloriecountercharts.com. Mike Vincitorio. January 2010

www.indoorclimbing.com/Protein_Food.html

Index

www.ingramcontent.com/pod-product-compliance
Lightning Source LLC
Chambersburg PA
CBHW072022080426
42733CB00010B/1795